In Situ Hybridization Protocols for the Brain

BIOLOGICAL TECHNIQUES

A Series of Practical Guides to New Methods in Modern Biology

Series Editor

DAVID B SATTELLE

Computer Analysis of Electrophysiological Signals
J Dempster
Fluorescent and Luminescent Probes for Biological Activity
WT Mason (Editor) (published May 1993)
Planar Lipid Bilayers
W Hanke and W-R Schlue (published October 1993)

CLASSIC TITLES IN THE SERIES

Microelectrode Methods for Intracellular Recording and Ionophoresis
RD Purves
Immunochemical Methods in Cell and Molecular Biology
RJ Mayer and JH Walker

BIOLOGICAL TECHNIQUES

In Situ Hybridization Protocols for the Brain

Edited by

W. WISDEN   and   B.J. MORRIS

MRC Laboratory
of Molecular Biology,
Cambridge, UK

Department of Pharmacology,
University of Glasgow,
Glasgow, UK

ACADEMIC PRESS
Harcourt Brace & Company, Publishers
London · San Diego · New York
Boston · Sydney · Tokyo · Toronto

ACADEMIC PRESS LIMITED
24–28 Oval Road
London NW1 7DX

United States Edition published by
ACADEMIC PRESS INC.
San Diego, CA 92101

Copyright © 1994 by
ACADEMIC PRESS LIMITED

This book is printed on acid-free paper

A catalogue record for this book is available from the British Library

ISBN 0–12–759919–3 (hardback)
ISBN 0–12–759920–7 (bench-top edition)

Typeset by J&L Composition Ltd, Filey, North Yorkshire
Printed and bound in Great Britain at The Bath Press, Avon

Series preface

The rate at which a particular aspect of modern biology is advancing can be gauged, to a large extent, by the range of techniques that can be applied successfully to its central questions. When a novel technique first emerges, it is only accessible to those involved in its development. As the new method starts to become more widely appreciated, and therefore adopted by scientists with a diversity of backgrounds, there is a demand for a clear, concise, authoritative volume to disseminate the essential practical details.

Biological Techniques is a series of volumes aimed at introducing to a wide audience the latest advances in methodology. The pitfalls and problems of new techniques are given due consideration, as are those small but vital details that are not always explicit in the methods sections of journal papers. The books will be of value to advanced researchers and graduate students seeking to learn and apply new techniques, and will be useful to teachers of advanced undergraduate courses, especially those involving practical and/or project work.

When the series first began under the editorship of Dr John E Treherne and Dr Philip H Rubery, many of the titles were in fields such as physiological monitoring, immunology, biochemistry and ecology. In recent years, most biological laboratories have been invaded by computers and a wealth of new DNA technology. This is reflected in the titles that will appear as the series is relaunched, with volumes covering topics such as computer analysis of electrophysiological signals, planar lipid bilayers, optical probes in cell and molecular biology, gene expression, and *in situ* hybridization. Titles will nevertheless continue to appear in more established fields as technical developments are made.

As leading authorities in their chosen field, authors are often surprised on being approached to write about topics that to them are second nature. It is fortunate for the rest of us that they have been persuaded to do so. I am pleased to have this opportunity to thank all authors in the series for their contributions and their excellent co-operation.

DAVID B SATTELLE ScD

Acknowledgements

We are indebted to the Series Editor, Dr David Sattelle (Zoology Department, Cambridge University) for giving us the opportunity to assemble this book. Most importantly, we thank all our colleagues and friends for their willingness to contribute and promptly write their chapters. Finally, we are very grateful to the Commissioning Editor, Dr Carey Chapman (Academic Press, London) for important advice and input on all things editorial. We thank Oxford University Press for permission to cite from 'Theories of Everything', by John D. Barrow (OUP, 1991).

Bill Wisden
Brian Morris
September 1993

Contributors

S.J. Augood *MRC Molecular Neuroscience Group, Dept of Neurobiology, AFRC Babraham Institute, Babraham, Cambridge CB2 4AT, UK*

P.C. Emson. *MRC Molecular Neuroscience Group, Dept of Neurobiology, AFRC Babraham Institute, Babraham, Cambridge CB2 4AT, UK*

C. De Felipe *MRC Laboratory of Molecular Biology, MRC Centre, Hills Road, Cambridge CB2 2QH, UK*

B.R. Finsen *PharmaBiotec Research Center, Institute of Neurobiology, University of Aarhus, DK-8000 Aarhus C, Denmark*

A. Gerfin-Moser *Brain Research Institute, August-Forel Straße 1, CH-8029 Zurich, Switzerland*

A.L. Gundlach *University of Melbourne Clinical Pharmacology & Therapeutics Unit, Dept of Medicine, Austin and Repatriation Hospitals, Heidelberg, Victoria 3084, Australia*

B. Heppleman *Physiologisches Institut, Universität Würzburg, Röntgenring 9, D-8700 Würzburg, Germany*

S.P. Hunt *MRC Laboratory of Molecular Biology, MRC Centre, Hills Road, Cambridge CB2 2QH, UK*

D.J. Laurie *Centre for Molecular Biology (ZMBH), University of Heidelberg, Im Neuenheimer Feld 282, Heidelberg, D-69120, Germany*

E.M. McGowan *MRC Molecular Neuroscience Group, Dept of Neurobiology, AFRC Babraham Institute, Babraham, Cambridge CB2 4AT, UK*

L.A. McNaughton *MRC National Institute for Medical Research, The Ridgeway, Mill Hill, London NW7 1AA, UK*

H. Monyer *Centre for Molecular Biology (ZMBH), University of Heidelberg, Im Neuenheimer Feld 282, D69120 Heidelberg, Germany*

B.J. Morris   *Dept of Pharmacology, University of Glasgow, Glasgow G12 8QQ, UK*

R.D. O'Shea   *University of Melbourne Clinical Pharmacology & Therapeutics Unit, Dept of Medicine, Austin and Repatriation Hospitals, Heidelberg, Victoria 3084, Australia*

P.C.U. Schrotz   *Institute for Neurobiology, Im Neuenheimer Feld 364, University of Heidelberg, Heidelberg, D-6900 Germany*

D.J.S. Sirinathsinghji   *Merck, Sharp and Dohme Research Laboratories, Neuroscience Research Centre, Terlings Park, Eastwick Road, Harlow, Essex CM20 2QR, UK*

A. Ultsch   *BASF Ltd, Abt. Biotechnology, Carl-Bosch-Str. 38, D-67056, Ludwigshafen, Germany*

P. Wahle   *Ruhr-Universität Bochum, Fakultät für Biologie, Lehrtuhl für Allgemeine Zoologie und Neurobiologie, Universitäts Strasse 150, ND 7/31, Postfach 10 21 48, D-44780 Bochum 1, Germany*

W. Wisden   *MRC Laboratory of Molecular Biology, Neurobiology Division, MRC Centre, Hills Road, Cambridge CB2 2QH, UK*

Contents

PART II
Non-radioactive *in situ* Hybridization Methods

CHAPTER EIGHT
Non-radioactive *in situ* Hybridization using Alkaline Phosphatase-Labelled
Oligonucleotides   **81**
S.J. Augood, E.M. McGowan, B.R. Finsen, B. Heppelman and P.C. Emson

CHAPTER NINE
Combining Non-radioactive *in situ* Hybridization with Immunohistological and
Anatomical Techniques   **98**
P. Wahle

CHAPTER TEN
***Drosophila* Central Nervous System – Non-radioactive *in situ* Hybridization using**
Wholemounts   **121**
A. Ultsch

Colour plates are located between pages   84–85

Introduction: studying gene expression in neural tissues by *in situ* hybridization

W. WISDEN & B.J. MORRIS

GENERAL INTRODUCTORY REMARKS

In situ hybridization (ISH) is an important method for tracing the regional and cellular sites of gene expression within a tissue (Gee *et al.*, 1983). It is a particularly valuable tool when applied to the brain, because it allows the specific cell types expressing a given gene to be delineated from the complex mosaic of other cells constituting neuronal tissue. As a consequence, the ISH procedure often gives very striking and sometimes beautiful images.

The essence of the technique is simple. A nucleic acid probe, tagged with either radiolabelled nucleotides or other molecules allowing colorimetric/light detection, is hybridized directly to a tissue section, where it recognizes its cognate mRNA and forms a probe–mRNA duplex. After the excess probe has been washed away, the section is either exposed for autoradiography or processed histochemically to reveal the sites on the section targeted by the probe. Unfortunately, this simple scheme can be marred by excessively complex methodology and we hope that the first part of this book will serve as a corrective to this and show just how simple the method can be.

WHY ANOTHER BOOK ON *IN SITU* HYBRIDIZATION?

Why yet another book on this method? In some senses, the topic has already been covered in depth by some scholarly precursors (Uhl, 1987; Conn, 1989; Chesselet, 1990; Polak & McGee, 1990; Wilkinson, 1992), and is obviously a very widely used method available to many laboratories. Nevertheless, with the field of molecular neurobiology rapidly proliferating (*Cold Spring Harbour Symposia on Quantitative Biology, LV, The Brain*, 1990), there are still many people we have met who would like to set up the method and want a nice simple protocol. However, a glance through the currently available manuals reveals,

IN SITU HYBRIDIZATION PROTOCOLS FOR THE BRAIN
ISBN 0–12–759919–3

in our opinion, the problem – there are just too many different methods to choose from (e.g. oligonucleotides, cRNA probes, cDNA probes). Each protagonist has their own idiosyncratic approaches, and it is difficult to know what is important and what has been untested. Even similar sorts of methods (e.g. using oligonucleotides) sometimes employ widely differing approaches in the same book (Conn, 1989), and do not always appear to have been optimized. Nevertheless, it seems clear that oligonucleotides, the use of which has been developed and popularized particularly by Young and collaborators at NIH (Young *et al.*, 1986a,b) and Watson and colleagues (Lewis *et al.*, 1985) offer the simplest and quickest option. In this book we have therefore made a deliberate decision not to describe methods based on using cRNA/cDNA probes except for some special instances involving non-radioactive labelling (see Chapters 9 and 10) where such probes may be more sensitive.

Our own offering aims to present an integrated and (hopefully) streamlined/minimalist approach which would be suited to both large-scale projects and those involving characterization of transcription patterns of newly isolated genes. The first part of the book (Chapters 1–7) is a kind of 'family affair' based on the single application of a modified version of the Young and Lewis method using radiolabelled oligonucleotides (Lewis *et al.*, 1985; Young *et al.*, 1986a,b; Wisden *et al.*, 1991). However, since publishing our original protocol (Wisden *et al.*, 1991), it has undergone further significant improvements. Chapter 1 describes the method in detail using rat brain sections as a model system. All the authors in Chapters 2–6 then discuss modifications of the *same* protocol (e.g. with respect to producing high-quality embryo sections, logistics of large tissue specimens, processing neuronal/glial cell cultures for *in situ* hybridization, adapting it for roller cultures or studying insect nervous systems). This mode of presentation has two advantages: (i) repetition is avoided, because methods such as probe labelling, hybridization, etc., are carried out identically with that described in Chapter 1; (ii) as we know all the people involved, we can personally vouch that all of the applications in Chapters 1–7 actually work!

The essentials of our current protocol in Chapter 1 originally evolved in Dr Stephen Hunt's laboratory at the Medical Research Council Centre in Cambridge (Wisden *et al.*, 1991) and the contributors in Chapters 2–7 represent a network of people who either came to the Hunt laboratory to learn it, or learnt it from other people who had been there. The result has been that many research groups working on diverse topics are now using it successfully. The current track record is as follows: (i) neurotransmitter receptors, e.g. for γ-aminobutyric acid (GABA), glycine, glutamate (AMPA, high-affinity kainate, NMDA), nicotinic acetylcholine, 5-hydroxytryptamine (5-HT) and cannabinoids (Wisden *et al.*, 1988; Morris *et al.*, 1990; Sommer *et al.*, 1990; Malosio *et al.*, 1991; Voigt *et al.*, 1991; Monyer *et al.*, 1992; Munro *et al.*, 1993); (ii) neuropeptides, e.g. NPY, galanin, enkephalin (Morris, 1989; Gundlach *et al.*, 1990; Sirinathsinghji *et al.*, 1990); (iii) vesicle components (Marqueze-Pouey *et al.*, 1991); (iv) kinases (Thomas and Hunt, 1993); (v) transcription factors (Wisden *et al.*, 1990; McNaughton & Hunt, 1992; Rutherford *et al.*, 1992).

ADVANTAGES OF THE RADIOLABELLED-OLIGONUCLEOTIDE METHOD OF CHAPTER 1

(1) Little time or molecular biology experience needed

Very little hands-on time is needed. Virtually no molecular biology expertise is required. People to whom we have demonstrated the method described in Chapter 1 have always been pleasantly surprised to learn how simple and 'low tech' it actually is, and they have been able to set it up very quickly in their own laboratories. For example, it is certainly much simpler than immunocytochemistry and, in a large laboratory, can be performed almost on a routine/technical support basis much as any other molecular biological method. It certainly need not take up your full energies. In our hands the method gives comparable results to the best obtained with cRNA or cDNA probes.

(2) High throughput

Large numbers of oligonucleotide probes (e.g. up to 20 at one time) and sections can be handled at once. The method is very well suited to relatively large-scale mapping studies that involve comparing the expression of all known members of a particular gene family in the brain (e.g. see Laurie *et al.*, 1992; Wisden *et al.*, 1992; Tölle *et al.*, 1993). In our opinion much more effort and time is required to do similar sorts of things with cRNA/cDNA probes, or even with some other currently used oligonucleotide approaches.

The 1990s will see us flooded with sequence data generated from the Human Genome Project (Watson, 1990). Related projects are also underway involving comprehensive sequence tagging to identify all mRNAs found in brain (Adams *et al.*, 1993). Thus there will be a growing need to characterize the transcription pattern of these new genes. Although methods not dependent on prior knowledge of cDNA sequence have also been suggested using single stranded DNA probes derived from m13 phage (Boehm *et al.*, 1991), we believe an oligonucleotide based approach, particularly with respect to known sequences, will be the most economical in terms of bench hours.

(3) mRNA splice variants

Oligonucleotides are the only practicable method of distinguishing between mRNAs differing in only very small regions of nucleotide sequence. For example, the Chapter 1 method has been employed to study the Flip and Flop versions of AMPA/glutamate receptor mRNAs in rat brain (Sommer *et al.*, 1990) and two variants of the $\gamma2$ subunit of the $GABA_A$ receptor mRNA in the chick brain (Glencorse *et al.*, 1992).

MODIFICATION OF BASIC OLIGONUCLEOTIDE METHOD (CHAPTERS 2 TO 6)

As far as we are aware, the protocol given in Chapter 1 appears to be the simplest method available for the use of oligonucleotides for *in situ* hybridization. However, some modifications are necessary when the method is used for particular applications and these are described by authors who have direct experience of these techniques in Chapters 2–6. The problems presented by embryonic and neonatal tissue, or comparatively large tissue sections, are described in Chapters 2 and 3 respectively. In Chapter 4, Linda McNaughton *et al.* present the adaptation of the method for measuring mRNA levels in individual cultured cells (both neuronal and glial), while Chapter 5 (Gerfin-Moser and Monyer) shows the potential for applying *in situ* hybridization technology to organotypic cultures. Chapter 6 describes an extension of the basic method as used to study *Drosophila* tissues (Ultsch *et al.*, 1991). Although non-radioactive methods seem to have largely taken over for the study of young embryonic tissue, because of the ease of using wholemounts (Tautz & Pfeifle, 1989; Rosen & Beddington, 1993; see Chapter 10), older and adult tissues still have to be sectioned in the traditional manner. Chapter 6 shows that the battery of pretreatments of sections before hybridization normally used by researchers studying *Drosophila* can be omitted. The modifications detailed here should be of use to neuroscientists working with invertebrates in general.

Finally, Chapter 7 (O'Shea and Gundlach) covers the principles of a very important feature of *in situ* hybridization studies – the ability to quantify the signal and detect alterations in mRNA levels in response to physiological stimuli.

PART II: NON-RADIOACTIVE METHODS

The second half of this book is directed towards more recent and less standardized advances in *in situ* hybridization technology. These methods are currently much less used, possibly because they may be less sensitive than radioactive methods and also because they obviously require more finesse and general fiddling around to get them to work. However, once up and running, they have the advantage of high speed, giving a signal with cellular resolution within 2 days of the start of the experiment. Further, many will be keen to co-localize mRNA and protein within the same cell, and non-radioactive techniques are invaluable when any type of double-labelling is required. Dr. Piers Emson's laboratory has been one of the pioneers of non-radioactive approaches employing oligonucleotides conjugated to alkaline phosphatase (e.g. Kiyama & Emson, 1990; Kiyama *et al.*, 1991) and their detailed protocol is given in Chapter 8. The simultaneous use of antibodies and digoxygenin-labelled cRNA probes (Boeringher-Mannheim system, see *Non-radioactive In Situ Hybridization Application Manual* from Boeringher-Mannheim) sometimes combined with tract-tracing is discussed by Wahle (Wahle and Beckh, 1992; Wahle, Chapter 9). As described by Ultsch (Chapter 10), non-radioactive approaches (again using the Boeringher-Mannheim digoxygenin system) are particularly well established for the *Drosophila* embryo nervous system. As first shown by Tautz & Pfeifle (1989), no sectioning of embryos is required, as they are sufficiently small to permit the use of whole-mounts. Future developments are likely to see the increasing use of wholemounts to study gene expression in vertebrate development (Rosen & Beddington, 1993).

It is our experience, and that of the other authors who have kindly agreed to contribute chapters, that *in situ* hybridization techniques can be used in any laboratory by anyone. We are certain that even people already using *in situ* hybridization on a routine basis will find some of the advice given in these chapters useful. However, this book has been designed so that someone without any previous experience of the techniques can follow the recipes and expect to get a good result. Our advice is simple – have a go!

REFERENCES

Adams, M.D., Kerlavage, A.R., Fields, C. & Venter, J.C. (1993) *Nature Genet.* **4**, 256–267.

Boehm, T., Gonzalez-Sarmiento, Kennedy, M. & Rabbitts, T.H. (1991) *Proc. Natl. Acad. Sci. USA* **88**, 3927–3931.

Chesselet, M.-F. (1990) *In situ hybridization histochemistry*. CRC Press, Ann Arbor and Boston.

Conn, P.M. (ed.) (1989) *Gene probes. Methods in neurosciences*. Vol. 1. Academic Press, London.

Gee, C.E., Chen, C.L., Roberts, J.L., Thompson, R. & Watson, S.J. (1983). *Nature* **306**, 374–376.

Glencorse, T.A., Bateson, A.N. & Darlison, M.G. (1992) *Eur. J. Neurosci.* **4**, 271–277.

Gundlach, A.L., Wisden, W., Morris, B.J. & Hunt, S.P. (1990) *Neurosci. Lett.* **114**, 241–247.

Kiyama H. & Emson, P.C. (1990) *Neuroscience* **38**, 223–244.

Kiyama H., McGowan E.M. & Emson, P.C. (1991) *Mol. Brain Res.* **9**, 87–93.

Laurie, D.J., Seeburg, P.H. & Wisden, W. (1992) *J. Neurosci.* **12**, 1062–1087.

Lewis, M.E., Sherman, T.G. & Watson, S.J. (1985) *Peptides* **6**, Suppl. 2, 75–87.

Malosio, M.L., Marqueze, Pouey, B., Kuhse, J. & Betz, H. (1991) *EMBO J.* **10**, 2401–2409.

Marqueze-Pouey, B., Wisden, W., Malosio, M.L. & Betz, H. (1991) *J. Neurosci.* **11**, 3388–3397.

McNaughton, L.A. & Hunt, S.P. (1992) *Mol. Brain Res.* **16**, 261–266.

Monyer, H., Sprengel, R., Schoepfer, R., Herb, A., Higuchi, M., Lomeli, H., Burnashev, N., Sakmann, B. & Seeburg, P.H. (1992) *Science* **256**, 1217–1221.

Morris, B.J. (1989) *J. Comp. Neurol.* **290**, 358–368.

Morris, B.J., Hicks, A.A., Wisden, W., Darlison, M.G., Hunt, S.P. & Barnard, E.A. (1990) *Mol. Brain Res.* **7**, 305–315.

Munro S., Thomas, K.L. & Abu-Shaar, M. (1993) *Nature* **365**, 61–65.

Polak, J.M. & McGee, J.O'D. (eds.) (1990) *In situ hybridization. Principles and practice*. Oxford University Press, Oxford.

Rosen, B. & Beddington, R.S.P. (1993) *Trends Genet.* **9**, 162–167.

Rutherfurd, S.D., Widdop, R.E., Sannajust, F., Louis, W.J. & Gundlach, A.L. (1992) *Mol. Brain Res.* **13**, 301–312.

Sirinathsinghji, D.J.S., Morris, B.J., Wisden, W., Northrop, A., Dunnett, S.P. & Hunt, S.P. (1990) *Neuroscience* **34**, 675–686.

Sommer, B., Keinänen, K., Verdoorn, T.A., Wisden, W., Burnashev, N., Herb, A., Köhler, M., Takagi, T., Sakmann, B. & Seeburg, P.H. (1990) *Science* **249**, 1580–1585.

Tautz, D. & Pfeifle, C. (1989) *Chromosoma* **98**, 81–85.

Thomas, K.L. & Hunt, S.P. (1993) *Neuroscience* **56**, 741–757.

Tölle, TR., Berthele, A., Zieglgänsberger, W., Seeburg, P.H. & Wisden, W. (1993) *J. Neurosci.* (in press).

Uhl, G.R. (ed.) (1987) *In situ hybridization in brain.* Plenum Press, New York.

Ultsch, A., Schuster, C.M., Betz, H. & Wisden, W. (1991). *Nucleic Acids Res.* **19**, 3746.

Voigt, M.M., Laurie, D.J., Seeburg, P.H. & Bach, A. (1991) *EMBO J.* **10**, 4017–4023.

Wahle. P. & Beckh, S. (1992) *J. Neurosci. Methods* **41**, 153–166.

Watson, J.D. (1990) *Science* **248**, 44–48.

Wilkinson, D. (ed.) (1992) *In situ hybridization – A practical approach.* Oxford University Press/IRL Press, Oxford.

Wisden, W., Morris, B.J., Darlison, G., Hunt, S.P. & Barnard, E.A. (1988) *Neuron* **1**, 937–947.

Wisden, W., Errington, M.L., Williams, S., Dunnett, S.B., Waters, C., Hitchcock, D., Evan, G., Bliss, T.V.P. & Hunt, S.P. (1990) *Neuron* **4**, 603–614.

Wisden, W., Morris, B.J. & Hunt, S.P. (1991) In: *Molecular neurobiology: a practical approach*, J. Chad and H. Wheal (eds) Oxford University Press/IRL Press, Oxford. pp. 205–225.

Wisden, W., Laurie, D.J., Monyer, H. & Seeburg, P.H. (1992) *J. Neurosci.* **12**, 1040–1062.

Young, W.S. III, Bonner, T.I. & Brann, M.R. (1986a) *Proc. Natl. Acad. Sci. USA* **83**, 9827–9831.

Young, W.S. III, Mezey, E. & Siegel, R.E. (1986b) *Mol. Brain Res.* **1**, 231–241.

PART I

In Situ Hybridization with ³⁵S-Labelled Oligonucleotide Probes

CHAPTER ONE

In situ hybridization with synthetic oligonucleotide probes

W. WISDEN* and B.J. MORRIS†

* MRC Laboratory of Molecular Biology, Neurobiology Division, MRC Centre, Hills Road, Cambridge CB2 2QH, UK
† Department of Pharmacology, University of Glasgow, Glasgow G12 8QQ, UK

1.1 INTRODUCTION: mRNA HYBRIDIZATION USING SYNTHETIC OLIGODEOXYRIBONUCLEOTIDE PROBES

'Science is most at home attacking problems that require technique rather than insight. By technique we mean the systematic application of a sequential procedure – a recipe.' John D. Barrow. *Theories of Everything.*

Before reading this chapter, please read the Introduction (page 1).

In situ hybridization (ISH) to brain-derived tissue using synthetic oligonucleotides was largely developed and popularized by Young and collaborators and Lewis and collaborators (Lewis *et al.*, 1985, 1988; Young *et al.*, 1986a,b; Young, 1989). There are many variations of their method (e.g. Wisden *et al.*, 1991b), but the protocol we present here is possibly the simplest one published to date. ISH with oligonucleotides is an extremely straightforward procedure. The basic scheme is summarized in Figure 1.1. Slide-mounted sections are cut from unfixed frozen tissue in the standard histological manner on a cryostat. Sections are then lightly fixed and stored in ethanol at 4°C until required (Section 1.2). Oligonucleotides (Section 1.3) are radio-labelled (tailed) using terminal deoxyribonucleotide transferase and 'hot' deoxyadenosine triphosphate (usually $[\alpha\text{-}^{35}S]dATP$). The labelling reaction is described in Sections 1.3.1 and 1.3.2. Once the probes are labelled, they are diluted in hybridization buffer (Section 1.4), and the probe/hybridization buffer mix is applied to a processed brain section (Section 1.4), and hybridized overnight. The next day, excess probe is washed off, and after dehydration the sections can be exposed to either X-ray film to produce a global image (Section 1.5) or dipped in photographic emulsion for cellular resolution (Section 1.6). The recent commercial availability of $[\alpha\text{-}^{33}P]dATP$ (Zagursky *et al.*, 1991) might be of value for further

IN SITU HYBRIDIZATION PROTOCOLS FOR THE BRAIN
ISBN 0–12–759919–3

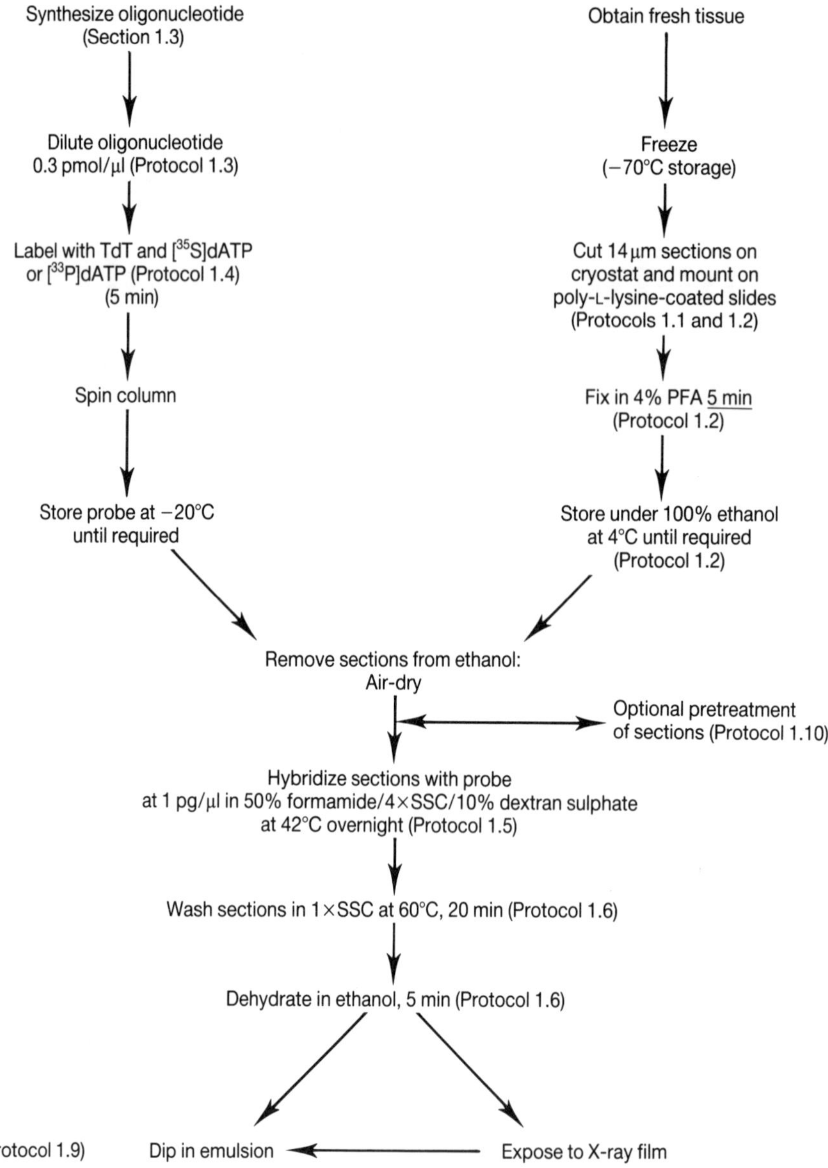

Figure 1.1 Schematic outline of the *in situ* hybridization method used in this chapter. Note that Protocol 1.10 (pretreatment of sections) need generally only be used for the adrenal gland, retina and possibly some embryo sections.

speeding up the ISH protocol when detecting very rare mRNAs (Section 1.3.5). β-electrons emitted from ^{33}P are approximately 1.5 times more energetic than those from ^{35}S. However, the resolution obtained with ^{33}P is roughly comparable, allowing exposure times to be reduced compared with those needed for ^{35}S (Section 1.3.5). The use of controls is discussed in Section 1.7 and the presentation of autoradiographs in Section 1.8.

1.1.1 ISH with oligonucleotides needs less 'hands-on' time than other methods (for the overall method, refer to Figure 1.1)

The advantages of using oligonucleotides are outlined in the Introduction. There is a lot of mythology connected with many aspects of the ISH method which add extra time constraints and expense, and which we have systematically

Protocol 1.1 Preparation of poly-L-lysine-coated slides.

1. Dissolve 25 mg of poly-L-lysine hydrobromide[a] in 5 ml of diethyl pyrocarbonate (DEPC)-treated water. Store as 1 ml aliquots at $-20°C$.
2. Thaw out one 1 ml tube of the 5 mg ml^{-1} aliquots of poly-L-lysine, and dilute it to 50 ml with DEPC-treated water, to give a 0.01% solution. Transfer this solution to a sterile 50 ml disposable plastic Petri dish.
3. Dip the baked slides[b] individually in the poly-L-lysine solution (immerse each slide completely), and allow slides to air-dry standing upright in a rack[c]. Slides can be stored for a few weeks at 4°C without any loss of adhesive properties.

[a] Poly-L-lysine hydrobromide, M_r 350 000 (Sigma, P-1524).
[b] A packet of standard 75 mm × 26 mm (e.g. BDH/Merck) microscope slides is wrapped in aluminium foil and baked (to sterilize them) for 4 h to overnight at 180°C. Slides are allowed to cool to room temperature before use. It is best to use slides that have a frosted edge so that they can easily be labelled with pencil. This is a better alternative than having to use a diamond pen.
[c] The type of rack used for standing slides upright is illustrated in the background of Figure 1.5, and simply consists of a piece of plastic (Perspex) plate with grooves cut across the surface to hold the bottom edges of the slides.

tried to remove. For example, we have found (Wisden *et al.*, 1991b), that pretreatments described in many protocols (e.g. proteinase K to increase probe access to mRNA, acetic anhydride to cover the section with negative charge to repel nucleic acids, and chloroform treatment to remove lipids which could also absorb nucleic acids non-specifically) are generally not needed for vertebrate brain and embryo sections hybridized with radiolabelled oligonucleotide probes. Similarly, prehybridization steps, whereby the section is preincubated with all of the hybridization buffer components except probe to absorb out non-specific binding sites, is also completely superfluous and can be eliminated. Furthermore, even many of the components in traditional hybridization buffers (salmon sperm DNA etc.) are unnecessary (see Section 1.4.1), as has also been reported by Lewis *et al.* (1988). However, certain types of tissue section (particularly those derived from retina and adrenal gland) may benefit from acetic anhydride/chloroform treatment (see Protocol 1.10).

1.2 PREPARATION OF SECTIONS (PROTOCOLS 1.1 AND 1.2)

At least in rodents and bovine samples, brain mRNA is stable for a remarkably long period

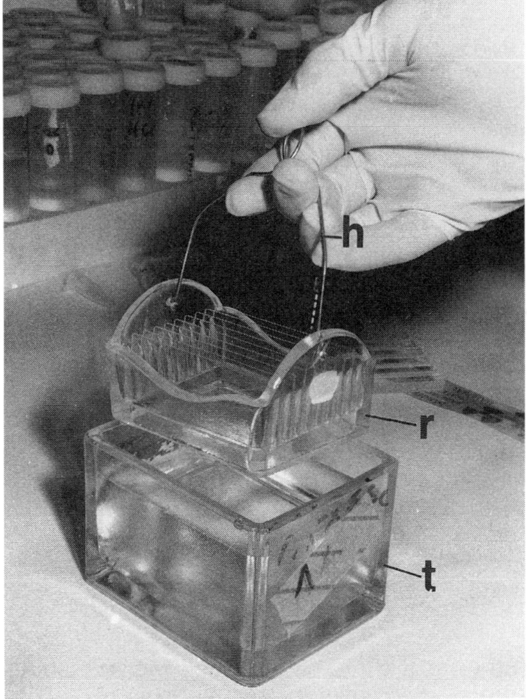

Figure 1.2 Illustration of the staining trough (t), slide rack (r) and wire handle (h) used for transferring the sections between different solutions (all detailed in the Histology section of the Laboratory Supplies Catalogue of BDH/Merck, 1993).

Protocol 1.2 Preparation and fixation of sections.

1. Cut 12–15 µm sections on a cryostat at −20°C. Thaw mount the sections on to poly-L-lysine-coated slides[a]. Allow sections to dry at room temperature for half an hour to several hours. For organizational purposes, slides can be consecutively numbered on their frosted area with pencil markings. Such pencil markings are effectively permanent. They do not come off in the ethanol storage or during hybridization/ washing steps. A frosted slide is illustrated in Figure 1.9.
2. Prepare a 4% solution of depolymerized paraformaldehyde (PFA) as follows. Transfer 40 g of paraformaldehyde[b] into 500 ml of sterile water. Heat the milky white suspension with continuous stirring until it reaches 60–65°C. Do not heat above this temperature. Carry out the whole procedure in a fume hood. Add 1.0 M NaOH dropwise until the suspension clears. Add 500 ml of 2 × PBS[c]. Mix well and chill the solution in an ice/water bath. Check that the pH is roughly 7.0. Best to use the same day.
3. Transfer a rack of dry sections into the ice-cold 4% PFA. Leave for 5 min[d].
4. Transfer sections into 1 × PBS[c] for several minutes. The exact time is not critical.
5. Transfer sections on to 70% ethanol[e] for several minutes.
6. Transfer the sections into the storage box[f] containing 95% or absolute ethanol. Store at 4°C in *cold room* until required. The storage of large quantities of 95% ethanol in refrigerators is not recommended because of the risk of ignition by sparking from thermostats. Note also that industrial grade ethanol (containing 5% methanol) works just as well as the more expensive pure grade. It is not critical whether 95% or absolute ethanol is used.

Glass staining troughs which hold 250 ml of solution (size: 93 × 75 × 55 mm internal) and matching glass racks with grooves (allowing transfer from one solution to another without removing the slides) are obtained from Merck Ltd/BDH. Stainless-steel wire handles for the glass racks are also available from BDH/Merck. These are listed in the Histology section of the Merck Laboratory Supplies Catalogue. Staining troughs and handles are illustrated in Figure 1.2.

[a] See Protocol 1.1 for the preparation of poly-L-lysine-coated slides.
[b] Paraformaldehyde (powder) is general-purpose reagent grade, e.g. Merck/BDH.
[c] 10 × PBS is 1.3 M NaCl, 70 mM Na_2HPO_4, 30 mM NaH_2PO_4. To make 1 litre of 10 × PBS, dissolve 75.79 g NaCl, 9.93 g Na_2HPO_4 anhydrous and 4.68 g $NaH_2PO_4.2H_2O$. Filter, treat with DEPC and autoclave. 2 × PBS and 1 × PBS are prepared by diluting the 10 × stock with sterile water.
[d] We use 19 slides/glass rack and 250 ml of solution in continental staining troughs. See Section 1.2 for details of glassware.
[e] Diluted from 100% ethanol with DEPC-treated water.
[f] Large plastic pizza boxes used for home freezing (e.g. a Stewart 'Seal Fresh' Pizza Storer, ref. 1225, UK) make convenient storage tanks for large numbers of rack (see Figure 1.3). Alternatively, sections can be stored in the continental staining troughs.

(up to at least 12 h) after death of the animal (Pittius *et al.*, 1985; Uhl *et al.*, 1985; Ross *et al.*, 1992), probably because before the breakdown and mixing of cellular compartments, RNAases may be largely separated from mRNA within the cell. Even 72 h *post mortem*, most rat brain RNA can be isolated intact (Ross *et al.*, 1992). Similar considerations seem to apply to post-mortem human brain, with post-mortem interval having at most only a modest effect on mRNA levels (e.g. Ross *et al.* (1992); reviewed extensively by Barton *et al.* (1993)). Emphasizing the stability

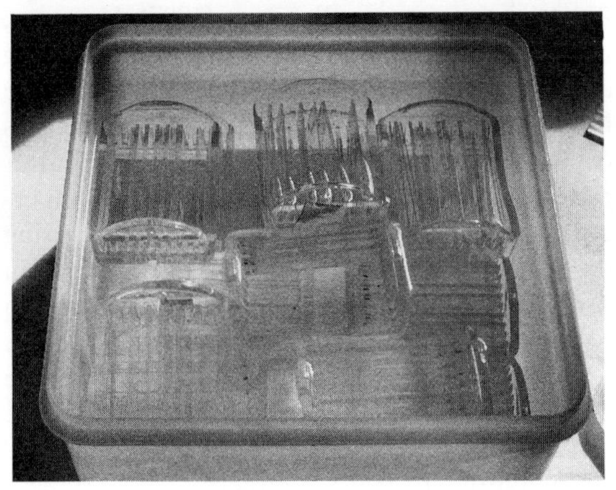

Figure 1.3 The storage of racks of sections under ethanol. A plastic/Tupperware box such as those used for home freezing (e.g. we use Stewart 'Seal Fresh' Pizza Storers, ref. 1225, UK) is filled with a couple of litres of absolute ethanol. Racks of slides are placed into the box, and then sealed with the lid (not shown) and placed into the *cold room*. IMPORTANT: Do *not* use refrigerators to store large quantities of flammable liquids.

of post-mortem RNA, Barton *et al.* observe that abundant intact biologically active RNA can still be found in human brain tissue which was not frozen until even 36 h after death, although they caution that the physiological state (e.g. hypoxia) of the patient before death may have adverse influences on certain RNAs. The conclusion is that if you wish to study qualitative patterns of gene expression, the post-mortem interval and manner of death may not be particularly critical, but for quantitative studies it is essential that type of death and post-mortem interval be matched as closely as possible (Barton *et al.*, 1993).

In practical terms, even if some degradation has occurred, it should not be a problem because mRNA need not be completely intact in order to be detected by ISH. This means that there is plenty of time for careful removal and dissection of the brain. We usually use non-perfused brains, although when using antibodies combined with ISH, cardiac perfused tissue is used (see, for example, Noguchi *et al.* (1991) and Chapter 9 of this volume). After removal of the unfixed brain, it is slowly frozen by placing it on a flat square of aluminium foil placed on top of powdered dry ice. Once it has been completely frozen (usually within 5–10 min), it can be wrapped in parafilm

(to prevent freeze-drying), placed in a poly-propylene screw-cap tube (e.g. 50 ml Falcon) and stored at −70°C (for months or years) until needed for cutting. After freezing, the tissue should *not* be allowed to thaw at any point as this may crack open the cells and allow RNAase access to RNA as well as destroying much of the cellular morphology. When freezing the brain, it should not be snap-frozen by dipping it into methanol/dry ice or liquid nitrogen as this shatters the tissue and makes it very difficult to cut good sections on the cryostat. On the day of cutting, the frozen material is transferred from the −70°C freezer to the −20°C cryostat chamber to equilibrate (for at least 1 h) before cutting. Sections are usually 15 μm thick (they can be thinner or thicker, depending on the applica-tion). When ^{32}P-labelled probes are used, thicker sections may give a higher signal as they contain more mRNA. Alternatively, very thin (5 μm) sections can be used for serially sectioning through large cells (e.g. motor neurons of the vertebrate spinal cord). This approach has been used to deduce coexpression of different γ-aminobutryric acid (GABA)$_A$ receptor subunit mRNAs in the same cell (Persohn *et al.*, 1992). Recently, Hökfelt's group have demonstrated that it is also possible to hybridize ^{35}S-labelled oligonucleotides to fresh unfixed sections, which could potentially further simplify the procedure for some applications (see Dagerlind *et al.*, 1992).

On the day of cutting, *fresh* 4% paraformalde-hyde (Protocol 1.2) and poly-L-lysine-coated slides are prepared (Protocol 1.1). Older solutions of paraformaldehyde may contain oxidation products which damage nucleic acids, although we sometimes use paraformaldehyde solutions that have been made up on the previous day. We have found poly-L-lysine to be the most effective substrate for ensuring section adhesion to slides for ISH. In our hands, sections never come off at high wash temperatures. The slide coating takes only 10 min for 50 slides (see Protocol 10.1), and once dry, they are ready to use. They can be stored for a limited period (for at least 1 week – some people store them for up to several months) at 4°C in sealed boxes.

For the cutting of vertebrate rat/mouse embryo sections and early postnatal sections, see Chapter 2. For the cutting of very large sections (e.g.

primate), see Chapter 3. For *Drosophila* sections, see Chapter 6.

1.2.1 Advantages of long-term storage of sections under ethanol

After cutting on a cryostat, most protocols indicate storage of sections desiccated at −70°C. In our experience, this is rather cumbersome. A certain degree of fastidiousness is required to label storage boxes, and it is difficult to see how many sections one actually has without unthawing the box. We have also had the impression that sections work les than optimally if they are freeze–thawed more than once. The storage of sections in 95% or absolute ethanol is far more versatile, principally because slides can be quickly removed from the ethanol for visual inspection and quickly replaced before they dry. The number of sections present and what they are can be seen clearly, and they can easily be reorganized or regrouped. Sections stored under ethanol are stable for long periods of time, at least as long as storage at −70°C, and large libraries of sections can be maintained. In our hands, sections stored for over 2 years in this way have shown no loss of signal. Once the sections have been removed from ethanol they are dry within minutes and are ready to be hybridized. In contrast, thawing out sections is time consuming and requires more rigid planning before the start of an experiment.

1.2.2 Sterility considerations

In our experience, ISH does not require *obsessive* precautions in preventing RNAse contamination. There is probably more RNAse in the tissue section than present in external sources. There is no need to use sterile equipment to remove the brain! However, if only for psychological security, it may be sensible to use (DEPC)-treated and autoclaved water to make up all the solutions used before the hybridization step and for the hybridization buffer itself, and also to wear gloves when handling reagents/slides before hybridization. For a useful and detailed consideration of the way to create a RNAse-free environment, see Blumberg (1987). However, it is very unlikely that any small contaminating quantities of RNAse will survive PFA, be active in the 100% ethanol used to store the sections or be very active in the hybridization buffer containing 50% formamide at elevated temperatures. The glassware used for fixing and rinsing the sections before ethanol storage is cleaned in a dishwasher but it is not found necessary to bake it. However, baked microscope slides are used before cutting (Protocol 1.1). After the hybridization step, there is no need to use sterile solutions, because of the resistance of DNA/RNA hybrids to RNAse attack.

1.3 OLIGONUCLEOTIDE PROBES: SYNTHESIS AND DESIGN

In a well-equipped molecular biology research institute, there will probably be a central facility devoted to oligonucleotide synthesis, probably using Applied Biosystems or Pharmacia machines. Alternatively, a glance through the classified sections of either *Nature* or *Science* reveals numerous companies/biochemistry departments (e.g. British Bio-Technology, Oxford, UK) offering to custom-build oligonucleotides to your specifications at competitive prices. One requires very small amounts of oligonucleotide for radioactive ISH experiments, with 0.3 pmol (approximately 5 ng of a 45-mer) of oligonucleotide being enough to hybridize 50 large horizontal rat brain sections. Consequently, one synthesis run of a particular oligonucleotide should be a lifetime's supply.

We usually find it unnecessary to purify oligonucleotides obtained from the synthesizers. Although the concentrated oligonucleotide solution (usually in the millimolar range) may look very dirty, when it is serially diluted to the low concentrations used for labelling (0.3 pmol μl^{-1}, see Protocol 1.3), any contaminants from the synthesis reaction do not seem to be a problem. A potential advantage in purifying an oligonucleotide by polyacrylamide gel electrophoresis (see Sambrook *et al.* (1989) for protocol) is that it will remove the many shorter polymer products present from the synthesizing reaction. However, in practice, these shorter forms do not seem to interfere with the ISH.

The original oligonucleotides used by Young seem to have been rather arbitrarily chosen as 48-mers (e.g. Young *et al.*, 1986a,b; Young, 1989). In practice, using the protocols in this chapter, one can use oligonucleotides anywhere in length from 36-mers (Sommer *et al.*, 1990) to 60-mers (Wisden *et al.*, 1990) using identical hybridization and wash conditions regardless of probe length. On a routine basis, we use 40- or 45-mers with basically no difference in results.

There are some simple guidelines for designing an oligonucleotide for use in hybridization studies (reviewed by Lewis *et al.*, 1988). In theory, if it is made from too many A or T residues, it may hybridize less efficiently because AT basepairs are relatively less stable than those of GC. Equally, it is probably not a good idea to build an oligonucleotide which is excessively GC-rich for the opposite reason, i.e. such a probe could give more non-specific binding. Thus, the probe should be designed such that the GC/AT ratio is between 50 and 65. It may also be possible that certain oligonucleotides can form hairpin structures and hybridize with themselves internally rather than with the target mRNA. In practice, it is advisable to follow an empirical approach. A sensible idea is to synthesize several oligonucleotides that will hybridize to different parts of the mRNA (see Section 1.7 on controls). If you feel sufficiently motivated, it may also be useful to run the intended sequence of your oligonucleotide against the EMBL/Genbank database to see if it is likely to hybridize to anything else. However, assuming that your probe does not recognize a unique mRNA splice variant, multiple oligo-nucleotides, which should give the same auto-radiographic pattern, serve as the best internal control (Section 1.7).

For investigators not so familiar with the conventions of molecular biology, note that published DNA sequences are usually given as the sense (coding or plus) strand, so that probes built to detect mRNA are constructed as comple-mentary sequence to this, and with the 5′ to 3′

Protocol 1.3 Dilution of oligonucleotides for ISH.

Typically, oligonucleotides arrive from our Applied Biosystems machines dissolved in TE (10 mM Tris, pH 7.0, 1 mM EDTA) buffer at around an average concentration of 1000 pmol μl^{-1} (i.e. 1 mM). A working stock solution used for TdT labelling is 0.3 pmol μl^{-1} (Protocol 1.2).
1. Take 10 µl of concentrated stock and dilute to 100 µl in sterile water (Dilution 1). (This (1/10) dilution can be kept as a permanent reserve of oligonucleotide stored at −20°C.) Also store the original synthesis stock at −20°C.
2. Take 5 µl of Dilution 1 (the 1/10 stock) and dilute to 1 ml in water (Dilution 2).
3. Measure the absorbance of the *total* 1 ml of Dilution 2 at 260 nm (A_{260}) with reference to sterile water as a blank.
   For an oligonucleotide, assume 1.0 A_{260} unit corresponds to 20 µg ml^{-1} (Sambrook *et al.*, 1989).
   For a 45-mer oligonucleotide, 0.3 pmol µl^{-1} is equivalent to 5 ng µl^{-1} (assuming average M_r of one nucleotide is 330).
4. Dilute the appropriate amount of oligonucleotide from Dilution 1 (the 1/10 dilution) into 1 ml of sterile water to give a working stock of 5 ng µl^{-1} (for a 45-mer).
This 5 ng µl^{-1} stock is stored at −20°C and can be freeze-thawed (*ad infinitum*) as required.
Specific example:
   For a particular 45-mer.
      5 µl of Dilution 1 in 1 ml of water gives A_{260} reading of 0.2.
      i.e. 5 µl of Dilution 1 contains 0.2 × 20 = 4 µg of oligonucleotide.
         Thus 1 µl of Dilution 1 contains 0.8 µg of oligonucleotide.
To prepare 1 ml of 5 ng µl^{-1} (0.3 pmol µl^{-1}) labelling stock, add 6.25 µl of Dilution 1 into 1 ml of water.

Protocol 1.4 Terminal transferase labelling reaction protocol.

For dilution of oligonucleotides, see Protocol 1.3.

In a standard labelling reaction, label 0.3 pmol of oligonucleotide (usually 45-mers) with 10 pmol of $[\alpha\text{-}^{35}S]$dATP or $[\alpha\text{-}^{33}P]$dATP, i.e. using a 30:1 molar ratio of isotope to oligonucleotide. This results in the addition of approximately 10–20 AMP residues to the 3′ end of the oligonucleotide (as assessed by polyacrylamide gel analysis). This small quantity of labelled oligonucleotide (0.3 pmol) is enough to hybridize 50 standard-size microscope slides (see the text).

Use terminal transferase (TdT 25 U μl^{-1}) from Boehringer-Mannheim. Reaction buffer (5×) (potassium cacodylate, 1 M, Tris/HCl, 125 mM, bovine serum albumin, 1.25 mg ml^{-1}, pH 6.6, at 25°C) and 25 mM $CoCl_2$ solution are supplied by the manufacturer with the enzyme. Store all components at -20°C and freeze–thaw as required.

For 10 µl volume (can be scaled up to 20 µl, just add double of everything, and add only 30 µl TE at the end):

1. Mix 1 µl of oligonucleotide at concentration of 0.3 pmol μl^{-1} (note that
for a 45-mer, 0.3 pmol is equivalent to 5 ng μl^{-1})
2 µl of 5 × reaction buffer (Boehringer-Mannheim)
0.6 µl of 25 mM $CoCl_2$ (Boehringer-Mannheim)
1.5 µl of $[\alpha\text{-}^{35}S]$dATP (1300 Ci $mmol^{-1}$, DuPont, NEN, NEG–034H)[a].
5 µl of sterile DEPC-treated water
1 µl of TdT at 25 U μl^{-1} (Boehringer-Mannheim)
2. Incubate for 5–8 min at 37°C. The exact labelling time may vary slightly depending on the batch of isotope or if a different supplier of enzyme is used. Certain enzyme brands require up to 1 h to achieve the same specific radioactivity.
3. Stop the reaction by adding 40 µl of TE buffer (10 mM Tris, 1 mM EDTA) or sterile water.
4. Apply the total 50 µl from step 3 to a Sephadex G-25 spin column (see Sambrook *et al.* (1989) for *exact* protocol) or to a commercial spin column (we use Bio-Spin 6 Columns from Bio-Rad laboratories, Richmond, CA 94804, USA). Spin at 2000 rpm for 2 min. This removes unincorporated nucleotides. The volume of the column eluate should be between 40 µl and 50 µl. Analyse 2 µl of the eluate by liquid-scintillation counting. The counts should be in the range 50 000 to 300 000 d.p.m. μl^{-1}. If counts are below the 50 000 d.p.m. μl^{-1} level, do not use the probe because the specific radioactivity is too low. If they are above 300 000 d.p.m. μl^{-1}, then in our experience, some non-specific binding may occur, probably because the AMP tail is too long. Counts for ^{33}P should also be at least 100 000–200 000 d.p.m. μl^{-1}. ^{33}P is also counted with scintillation liquid.
5. If the ^{35}S probe is OK, add 1 µl of 1 M DTT to the eluate[b]. This preserves the probe from oxidation. ^{33}P requires no DTT addition. Probes are stored at -20°C and can be freeze–thawed for repeated use. We use them for up to a month after labelling.

---

[a] For ^{33}P, use 10 pmol, i.e. 1 µl of $[\alpha\text{-}^{33}P]$dATP (1825 Ci $mmol^{-1}$, 10 µCi μl^{-1}, NEN, NEG -312H).
[b] DTT (dithiothreitol); 1 M stock; 3.09 g in 20 ml of sterile water. Store in 1 ml aliquots at -20°C. Freeze–thaw as required, but keep on ice.

polarity opposite to that of the sense strand. For example, if the sense strand sequence is 5'-GAATTCCCGGG . . . . . .3', then the sequence of the probe will be 5'-CCCGGGAATTC . . . . . .3'.

1.3.1 Probe labelling with terminal deoxynucleotidyl transferase (TdT) (Protocols 1.3 and 1.4)

ISH works best with a low probe concentration to reduce non-specific binding and hence requires high specific activity probes for optimal results. Thus for this purpose, oligonucleotides are labelled with terminal deoxynucleotidyl transferase (often called terminal transferase) which is a DNA polymerase that catalyzes the synthesis of polydeoxyribonucleotides from deoxyribonucleotide triphosphates with the release of inorganic pyrophosphate (reviewed in Sambrook *et al.* (1989) and Singer & Berg (1992)). It initiates the reaction from the free terminal 3'-hydroxyl group of single-stranded DNA, e.g. oligonucleotides. Thus, if [α-^{35}S]dATP, oligonucleotide and TdT are mixed, the end result is a polydeoxyadenylic (poly[^{35}S]dA) tail added to the 3' end of the oligonucleotide. The number of [^{35}S]dA residues added to the 3' end (which is directly proportional to the probe specific radioactivity) can be controlled by changing the molar ratio of [α-^{35}S]dATP to oligonucleotide. In our hands, a 30:1 molar ratio of [α-^{35}S]dATP to oligonucleotide is optimal. Longer tails tend to give high non-specific signals. Shorter tails require, of course, longer exposure times.

The TdT labelling method is given in Protocol 1.4. The TdT enzyme has unusual cofactor requirements (cobalt and potassium cacodylate), and so we find it more convenient to use a supplier (Boehringer-Mannheim) of the TdT enzyme that also supplies the reaction buffer, as preparation of the correct potassium cacodylate solution is tedious. If you want to prepare your own tailing buffer, then use the recipe exactly as described in Eschenfeldt *et al.* (1987).

To remove unincorporated nucleotides from the labelling reaction, we use commercially prepared spin columns (Biospin 6 from Bio-Rad) using the manufacturer's instructions. However, it is not much more effort to make and use Sephadex G-25 spin columns *exactly* as described in Sambrook *et al.* (1989). These work just as well as the commercial ones, and are a lot cheaper.

1.3.2 Logistics of labelling many probes simultaneously

One advantage of using oligonucleotides compared with other sorts of probes is that one can label many probes simultaneously because the number of operator steps is markedly less than those required to label a cRNA or an m13-derived probe. For example, in order to label ten oligonucleotides, it is most efficient to prepare a reaction cocktail containing reaction buffer, water, isotope and enzyme in order to minimize pipetting steps. In specific terms, for ten individual 10 µl reactions, 6 µl of CoCl$_2$, 20 µl of 5 × reaction buffer, 50 µl of sterile water, 15 µl of [α-^{35}S]dATP and 10 µl of TdT should be mixed in an Eppendorf tube on ice. This is, of course, simply the volume of each component in the reaction recipe given in Protocol 1.4 multiplied by 10. Mix by gentle vortexing. Centrifuge (brief pulse) to collect all the liquid to the bottom of the tube and pipette successively 10 µl of the cocktail on to 1 µl aliquots of each oligonucleotide (in separate tubes!) to start the reactions.

1.3.3 Storage of probes

After passage through the spin column, dithiothreitol (DTT) is added to stabilize ^{35}S probes (Protocol 1.4). The half-life of ^{35}S is approximately 3 months and probes can be stored at −20°C and freeze–thawed whenever they are needed. They can be used for at least up to 1 month after labelling and possibly longer. The half-life of ^{33}P is 29 days and probes can be similarly freeze–thawed and reused over this period. ^{33}P probes do not require DTT to stabilize them.

1.3.4 Trouble-shooting the TdT labelling reaction

Optimal counts after the spin column for ^{35}S-labelled probes are between 50 000 and

300 000 d.p.m. μl^{-1} from the 50 μl eluate. Although the TdT reaction usually works perfectly, sometimes it fails or works suboptimally (counts at or below 50 000 d.p.m. μl^{-1}). This is invariably found to depend on the batch of the isotope, which presumably contains impurities that inhibit the enzyme, although the manufacturers usually deny this. ^{35}S isotope reagents stabilized with DTT concentrations greater than 1 mM should not be used, otherwise DTT forms an insoluble complex with cacodylate in the reaction buffer and stops the enzyme activity. This used to be a frequent complaint about isotopes from Amersham, although this company now supplies a reformulated [α-^{35}S]dATP suitable for terminal transferase (Rattray and Priestley, 1993).

If the number of counts is below 50 000 d.p.m. μl^{-1}, the probe specific activity may be too low to detect moderately abundant or rare mRNAs, but it will still work for actin, tubulin and other extremely abundant mRNAs such as MAP-2. A remedy is to leave the reaction to incubate for a longer time, e.g. 30 min. In contrast, sometimes the reaction can work too well. Probes with counts in excess of 350 000–400 000 d.p.m. μl^{-1} may give some non-specific binding, particularly to granule cells of the vertebrate cerebellum (see Figure 1.12C) and other dense cell areas such as the hippocampus, probably because the poly(A) tail is too long. A shorter reaction time or only 1 μl of the [α-^{35}S]dATP instead of 1.5 μl should be tried (see Protocol 1.4). However, if the cerebellum or hippocampus is not required, such a probe may not be a problem and an autoradiographic signal will be obtained very quickly.

There seems to be considerable variation in enzyme activities depending on the supplier. For example, in our hands, the Boehringer-Mannheim enzyme requires only 5 min to achieve probes of the required specific radioactivity. Other sources of enzyme (e.g. Pharmacia) may require longer incubation periods (e.g. 30–60 min at 37°C) to achieve the same result.

1.3.5 ^{33}P-labelled probes

The E_{max} energy of emitted β-particles from ^{33}P is 0.25 MeV, whereas the β-particle E_{max} from

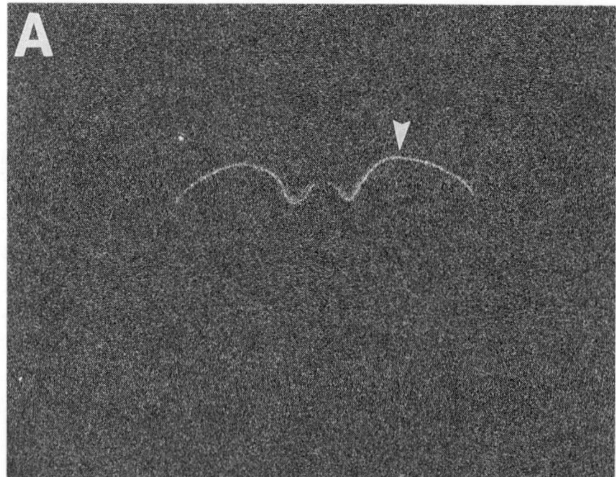
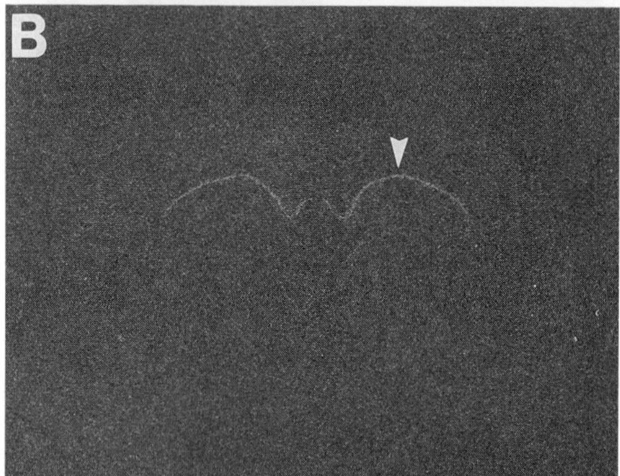
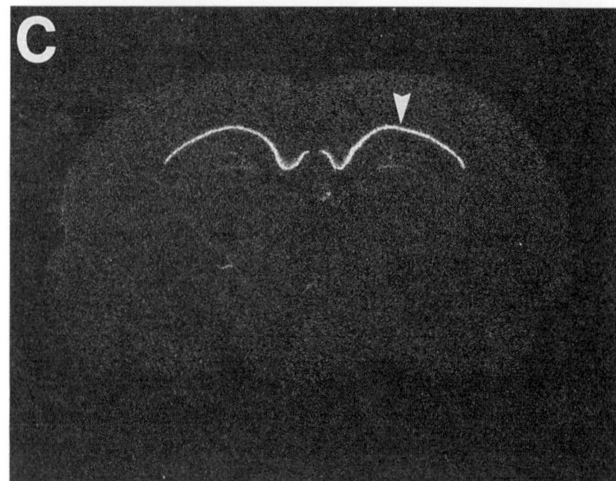

Figure 1.4 X-ray film (XAR-5) autoradiographs of coronal sections of adult rat brain demonstrating comparison between a poly[^{35}S]dA-labelled antisense oligonucleotide (A) and the same oligonucleotide tailed with poly[^{33}P]dA (B and C). The oligonucleotide hybridizes to an mRNA which is relatively specific for the CA1 pyramidal cells (arrowheads) of rat hippocampus (Erlander *et al.*, 1993; W. Wisden & M. Voigt, unpublished). See Section 1.3.5 for further details.

Protocol 1.5 Application and hybridization of probes to sections.

1. Remove the sections from 95% or absolute ethanol storage and allow to air-dry for anywhere between 5 min to half an hour. The exact time is not critical. Label the slides with the appropriate probe designation using a pencil on the frosted end of the slide. These pencil marks do not come off during any of the subsequent steps. If using sections of retina or adrenal gland, you may wish to pretreat the slides with acetic anhydride and/or chloroform before hybridization. If this is the case, transfer the sections straight from the 95% ethanol storage into 1 × PBS and go to step 2 of Protocol 1.10.
2. In an Eppendorf tube (for smaller volumes) or a 15 ml Falcon tube (for larger volumes), dilute the radiolabelled probe in hybridization buffer[a]. Because of the high viscosity of the hybridization buffer, the probe solution has a tendency to float immediately to the surface after addition to the hybridization buffer mix. Thus, it is very *important* to vortex the probe/hybridization buffer *vigorously* to achieve an even mix.
3. Apply 100 µl of probe/hybridization buffer to each slide[b]. If several sections are on each slide, make sure that there is some hybridization buffer on all the sections *before* putting on the parafilm.
4. Gently lower a parafilm coverslip over the drop of hybridization buffer (see Figure 1.4). The liquid should spread smoothly under the coverslip. Remove any large air bubbles by very gentle pressing with blunt-ended forceps, but any remaining small air bubbles are not a problem as they tend to disappear during the hybridization step[c].
5. To maintain humidity, saturate a small piece of tissue/filter paper with 50% formamide/4 × SSC[d] (where 1 × SSC is 0.15 M NaCl + 0.015 M sodium citrate, pH 7.0) and place this in the Petri dish[c] or Nunc Bio-Assay dish[c] as well (Figure 1.5). Place the lid tightly on the dish and incubate overnight at 42°C. It is advisable to further seal the lid of the dish by stretching layers of Parafilm around it.

[a] Probes are used at a very low concentration in the hybridization buffer. Dilute 1 µl (or 2 µl) of probe from the 50 µl spin column eluate into 100 µl hybridization buffer. Use 100 µl hybridization buffer/slide. Also add 1 µl of 1 M DTT 100 µl of hybridization buffer (however, this does not seem to do much because it can be missed out without any obvious difference to the result). Preparation of competition controls: Dilute the radiolabelled probe exactly as above but also add 2 µl of the corresponding unlabelled probe directly from the 0.3 pmol µl^{-1} stock for every 100 µl of hybridization buffer to generate a 100-fold excess of unlabelled probe.
[b] Use Parafilm 'M' laboratory film. American National Can TM., Greenwich, CT 06836, USA.
[c] Slides are laid horizontally in transparent plastic Petri dishes (for small numbers of slides) or Nunc Bio-Assay dishes (size: 243 × 243 × 18 mm) (for a large number of slides). If these dishes are placed on a black/dark surface, it becomes easy to see any air bubbles. Use parafilm strips cut to roughly 20 mm × 55 mm as coverslips. It is convenient to precut these before the experiment. Before use, remember to peel off the paper backing of the unexposed (virgin) side of the parafilm. Use this side to contact the hybridization liquid.
[d] We use a liquid for humidifying the hybridization chamber with essentially the same composition as the hybridization buffer to prevent any distillation between the two solutions.

^{35}S is 0.17 MeV (DuPont Biotech Update, 1992). Thus, exposures with ^{33}P to X-ray film should be roughly 1.5 times faster than those for ^{35}S for the same specific radioactivity, but the resolution on film is comparable. For very rare mRNAs, this may give ^{33}P a marginal edge. However, in our hands ^{35}S-labelled probes generally give superior results in terms of image quality.

Protocol 1.6 Washing sections after the hybridization.

All procedures can be non-sterile at this point.
1. Gently peel off the parafilm coverslips with blunt-ended forceps. Transfer the slides into 250 ml of 1 × SSC at room temperature. This step removes most of the unhybridized probe, before the higher stringency wash in step 2[a].
2. Transfer the rack of slides into 250 ml of prewarmed 1 × SSC at 60°C[b]. It is convenient to have the continental troughs in a 60°C water bath. Leave the sections washing for half an hour. The exact time is not critical. Agitation during washing is not required. Addition of DTT is also not required.
3. Transfer the rack through a brief (couple of seconds each) series of room temperature rinses in 1 × SSC, 0.1 × SSC[c], 70% ethanol, 95% ethanol (250 ml of each solution). Allow sections to air-dry (half an hour).
4. Expose sections to X-ray film or dip in emulsion (Protocol 1.9).

[a] Do not allow sections to dry after removal of coverslip, see Section 1.4.
[b] Many people use 1 × SSC at 55°C – it does not make any appreciable difference to the signal.
[c] 0.1 × SSC step is required to prevent salt precipitation on sections in ethanol.

Protocol 1.7 'Maximalist' oligonucleotide hybridization buffer.

The hybridization buffer is 50% formamide, 4 × SSC, 10% dextran sulphate, 5 × Denhardt's, 200 μg ml^{-1} acid–alkali-cleaved salmon sperm DNA, 100 μg ml^{-1} long-chain polyadenylic acid, 25 mM sodium phosphate, pH 7.0, 1 mM sodium pyrophosphate.

In a sterile graduated and screw-capped 50 ml polypropylene tube, add the following: 25 ml of 100% formamide[a], 10 ml of 20 × SSC[b], 2.5 ml of 0.5 M sodium phosphate, pH 7.0[c], 5 ml of 0.1 M sodium pyrophosphate, 5 ml of 50 × Denhardt's solution[d], 2.5 ml of 4 mg ml^{-1} acid–alkali-hydrolyzed salmon sperm DNA[e], 1 ml of 5 mg ml^{-1} polyadenylic acid[f] and 5 g of dextran sulphate[g]. After the dextran sulphate has dissolved, adjust to 50 ml with DEPC-treated water.

The dextran sulphate takes several hours, with occasional vortexing, to completely dissolve. It is best to place the tube on a rocker platform.

Store the hybridization buffer at 4°C in a sterile polypropylene (Falcon) tube. It keeps for at least 6 months and probably longer. Shake well before use. Do not boil the hybridization buffer before use.

[a] Use Fluka formamide. We have found that this brand requires no deionization before use. Use straight out of the stock bottle (stored at room temperature in light-tight bottle).
[b] 20 × SSC is 3 M NaCl, 0.3 M sodium citrate, pH 7.0, with HCl. Filtered, DEPC-treated and autoclaved. See Sambrook *et al.* (1989).
[c] 0.5 M sodium phosphate, pH 7.0, is prepared by mixing 0.5 M Na$_2$HPO$_4$ and 0.5 M NaH$_2$PO$_4$ until the pH reaches 7.0. The solution is then filtered, DEPC-treated and autoclaved.
[d] 50 × Denhardt's is 5 g of poly(vinylpyrrolidine), 5 g of bovine serum albumin (BSA), 5 g of Ficoll, 400–500 ml of DEPC-treated water. Store in aliquots at −20°C. See Sambrook *et al.* (1989)
[e] Prepared as described in Wisden *et al.* (1991b).
[f] Dissolve 100 mg of polyadenylic acid [5*], potassium salt (Sigma No. P-9403) in 20 ml of DEPC-treated water, to give 5 mg ml^{-1} stock. Store in 1 ml aliquots at −20°C.
[g] Dextran sulphate, sodium salt, molecular biology grade (Pharmacia).

Further, at the time of writing, ^{33}P is considerably more expensive than ^{35}S, so for us, ^{35}S remains the isotope of choice.

Figure 1.4 illustrates relative signal intensities of a probe tailed with poly ([^{35}S]dA) or poly ([^{33}P]dA) using a 30:1 molar ratio of dATP to oligonucleotide. The 45-mer probe hybridizes to an mRNA (encoding the serotonin (5-hydroxytryptamine) 5B receptor subtype) which is found predominantly in the CA1 sector of the rat hippocampus (Erlander *et al.*, 1993; W. Wisden & M. Voigt, unpublished work). The ^{35}S exposure (Figure 1.4A) was 4 weeks on XAR-5 X-ray film. Figure 1.4B illustrates the same oligonucleotide labelled with ^{33}P, with an exposure time of only 4 days. After 4 weeks on film, a saturated image results for the ^{33}P-labelled probe (Figure 1.4C). ^{33}P-labelled probes can also be used in emulsion studies for cellular resolution (e.g. see Lomeli *et al.*, 1993).

1.4 HYBRIDIZATION AND WASHING (PROTOCOLS 1.5 AND 1.6)

Once the probes have been labelled, and the sections cut and stored in ethanol, they can be hybridized at leisure. The probes are stable and can be reused (freeze–thawed) for at least a month and the sections are stable under ethanol for a very long time. The probe is diluted in the hybridization buffer to a concentration of 0.3 pmol/5000 µl (i.e. for a 45-mer, 1 pg µl^{-1}). This means 1 µl of the probe (from the 50 µl spin column eluate) per 100 µl of hybridization buffer. For a standard 25 mm × 75 mm microscope slide, 100 µl of hybridization buffer is needed after it has been spread out under a coverslip. Thus ten microscope slides require 1 ml of hybridization buffer and 10 µl of probe.

The hybridization buffer is prepared in large batches in 50 ml sterile polypropylene Falcon tubes (Protocol 1.7). This amount of buffer is enough for 500 standard slides. Hybridization buffer is stored in the tight-capped tube at 4°C, and is stable for a very long period (at least 6 months). With prolonged storage at 4°C, various components of the buffer described in Protocol 1.7 may precipitate out as a 'white smear', so

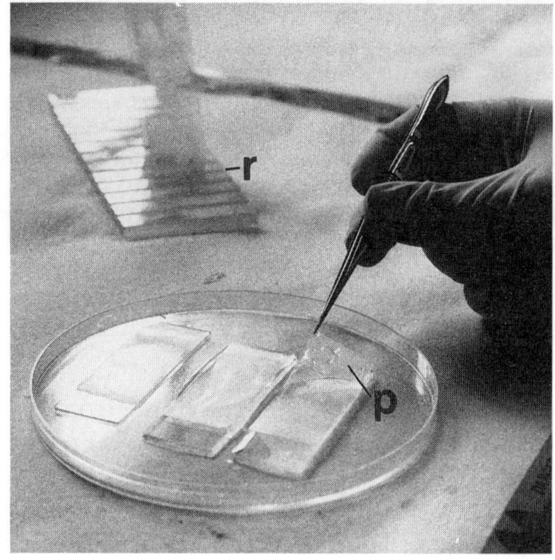

Figure 1.5 Parafilm (p) coverslips being placed over the hybridization mixture on slides. A perspex rack/plate (r) for holding the slides in an upright position is shown in the background (such a rack is also illustrated in the Microscope Slide Accessories section of the BDH/Merck Laboratory Supplies Catalogue, 1993).

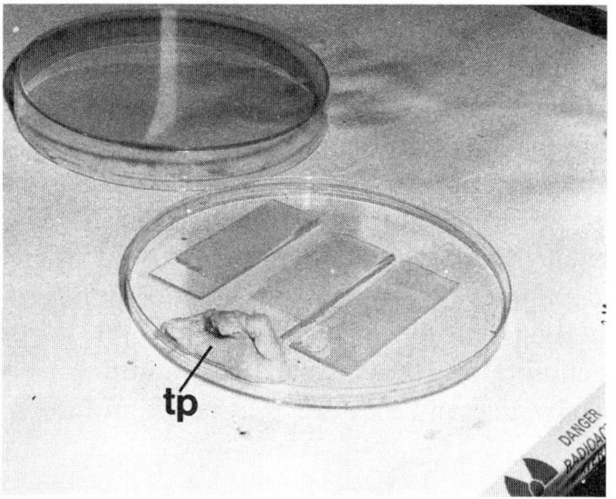

Figure 1.6 Illustration of a Petri dish hybridization chamber. A tissue paper (tp) saturated with 50% formamide/4 × SSC is shown in the Petri dish.

always shake/vortex the tube vigorously before use.

For the hybridization, use strips of parafilm (cut to about 20 mm × 55 mm) as coverslips to spread out the hybridization liquid (Protocol 1.5 and Figure 1.5). The hybridization chamber (usually a sealed plastic Petri dish) is kept moist

Protocol 1.8 'Minimalist' hybridization buffer.

The hybridization buffer is 50% formamide/4 × SSC/10% dextran sulphate. See also Protocol 1.7 for exact specifications of reagents.

In a sterile graduated and screw-capped 50 ml polypropylene tube, add 25 ml of 100% formamide (Fluka), 10 ml of 20 × SSC, sterile water to approx. 40 ml and 5 g of dextran sulphate. After dissolution (takes several hours with occasional vortexing, place on a rocker platform when not vortexing), adjust volume to 50 ml with sterile water.

Store at 4°C. Buffer is stable for at least 6 months and probably longer.

using a ball of tissue paper saturated in 50% formamide/4 × SSC (see Figure 1.6 and Protocol 1.5). Different people use different types of hybridization chamber. For a small number of slides, a sealed Petri dish is ideal (Figure 1.6). For larger numbers of slides, a nunc dish can be used (see Protocol 1.5, footnote c).

After hybridization, and before immersion of slides in wash solutions, the parafilm coverslips are pulled gently off the section with blunt-ended forceps, and the slides are then transferred directly into 1 × SSC solution at room temperature (Protocol 1.6). It is important not to allow the sections to dry between the removal of the coverslip and the immersion of the slide into the wash solution, otherwise the probe may become permanently 'baked' to the section with a subsequently terrible background. Thus, it is better to remove coverslips and transfer the slides *one at a time* into the washing buffer. For ^{35}S-labelled probes, most protocols suggest the use of 10 mM DTT or β-mercaptoethanol in the wash solutions to prevent coupling of ^{35}S to the section. However, we find their addition to be of no value and they are routinely omitted.

1.4.1. Components of the hybridization buffer; minimalist buffers (Protocol 1.8)

The key components of the hybridization buffer are formamide and Na^+ (in the form of SSC and dextran sulphate). Formamide makes it possible to lower the temperature at which hybridization occurs, thus preserving morphology. High salt concentrations promote hybridization rate, and dextran sulphate also serves to increase rate of hybridization (see Wahl *et al.* (1987) and

Sambrook *et al.* (1989) for reviews). Hybridization stringency is determined by temperature, percentage formamide and concentration of Na^+ ion. For a given hybridization temperature and length of oligonucleotide, a lower-percentage formamide mix corresponds to a lower stringency. In concrete terms, for a 45-mer hybridizing to mRNA, 50% formamide/4 × SSC at 42°C is considerably more stringent than 30% formamide/4 × SSC at 42°C. The latter might be more appropriate for a 26-mer (see Lathe (1985) and Albretsen *et al.* (1988) for a review of hybridization conditions for oligonucleotides used to target nucleic acids immobilized on membranes).

The other components of the hybridization buffer cocktail may prevent non-specific hybridization of probe to other RNAs or protein/lipid components in the section under certain conditions. They are designed to be present at such high concentrations that they compete with the probe for every non-specific site. For example, the polyadenylic acid is added to the hybridization buffer to compete with the polyadenylic tail of the probe. Similarly, salmon sperm DNA and Denhardt's solution are traditional nucleic acid-blocking reagents (see Sambrook *et al.*, 1989). Hydrolyzed salmon sperm DNA is used because it is already chemically broken into small pieces to lengths that compete more effectively with oligonucleotides. Pyrophosphate may compete with any remaining free nucleotides after the spin column, and sodium phosphate, pH 7.0, keeps the mix well buffered for optimal hybridization. Together, these components add to a collective overkill to prevent non-specific binding in a *maximal* hybridization buffer (Protocol 1.7).

However, all of these extra ingredients appear to be redundant in our current ISH system.

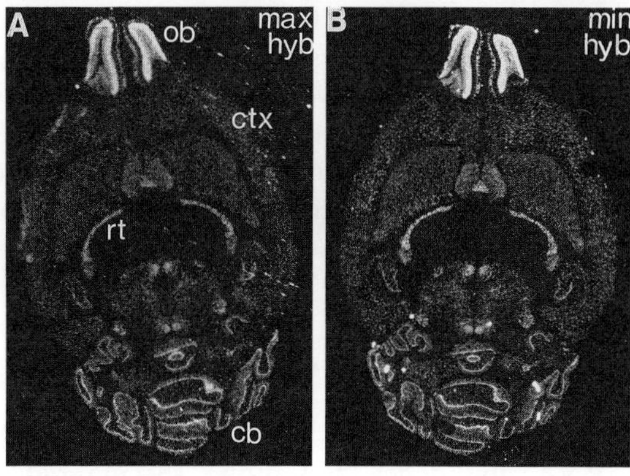

Figure 1.7 X-ray film autoradiographs of horizontal rat brain sections comparing the effects of hybridizing an ^{35}S-labelled antisense oligonucleotide recognizing the mRNA encoding rat glutamic acid decarboxylase in either (A) 'maximalist' buffer (Protocol 1.7) or (B) 'minimalist' buffer containing only formamide, SSC and dextran sulphate (Protocol 1.8). Exposure time was identical for both images (one week). cb, cerebellum; ctx, neocortex; ob, olfactory bulb; rt, reticular thalamic nucleus.

Figure 1.7 shows the results of an experiment in which an antisense 45-mer oligonucleotide designed to hybridize to the rat mRNA encoding glutamic acid decarboxylase was hybridized on parallel horizontal rat brain sections in two different hybridization buffers. The *minimalist* buffer contained only 50% formamide/4 × SSC/ 10% dextran sulphate (Figure 1.7B). The other buffer was the traditional *maximalist* hybridization buffer (Figure 1.7A). Thus, at the very low probe concentrations used in our ISH procedure, the minimalist buffer is just as effective as the traditional one, and therefore we now use the former on a routine basis.

1.4.2 Hybridization and post-hybridization washing conditions

The kinetics and efficiency of hybridization of oligonucleotides in solution to nitrocellulose-membrane-bound nucleic acids has been well studied (Lathe, 1985; Albretsen *et al.*, 1988). The length of the oligonucleotide and its nucleotide composition are critical parameters for determining optimal hybridization conditions. However, for ISH, where hybridization kinetics may

be quite different from those occurring on membranes, the predictive utility of these rules is of less value. An empirical approach works best. For example, when 36-mer oligonucleotides were used to distinguish between very closely related splice forms of glutamate receptor mRNAs (Sommer *et al.*, 1990), two of these probes (D Flop and A Flop) differed by only three of 36 nucleotides. Yet these probes largely gave different distributions in rat brain (Sommer *et al.*, 1990). So, clearly the hybridization conditions used in this experiment (50% formamide/ 4 × SSC/10% dextran sulphate at 42°C) combined with a low probe concentration are probably enough to achieve a distinction even with a three-nucleotide difference. Conversely, our conditions make it difficult to detect mRNAs during cross-hybridization between species, as a few dispersed nucleotide mismatches will drastically reduce efficiency of hybridization. Furthermore, for 36-mers, it essentially makes no difference to the qualitative autoradiographic pattern whether the sections are washed at 0.1 × SSC at 60°C (as in the original publication) or 1 × SSC at 60°C, except that the sections washed at higher stringency produce weaker signals overall. This again suggests that in this system, it is the stringency of the hybridization and not the washing conditions that may be the critical parameter in determining hybridization specificity.

1.5 EXPOSURE TO X-RAY FILM

After washing and dehydration (Protocol 1.6), slides are allowed to dry and are then ready to be exposed in a standard X-ray film cassette or dipped in liquid photographic emulsion (see Section 1.6). For vertebrate brains, to obtain a general global picture of the regions where a particular gene is expressed, to compare the distribution of different mRNAs and for ease of presentation (see Section 1.8), X-ray film resolution is usually the initial choice. For some regions of vertebrate brains and embryos, X-ray film alone is enough to determine which type or layer of cells is expressing the gene of interest. Even for sections as small as the rat spinal cord, X-ray film analysis can still provide useful

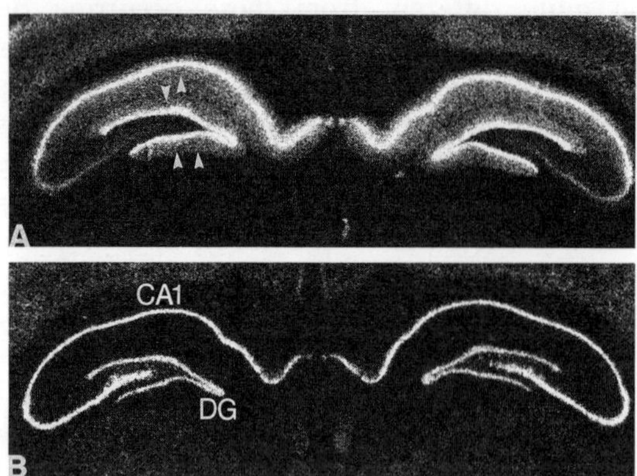

Figure 1.8 X-ray film (XAR-5) autoradiographs of coronal sections through the adult rat hippocampus from an ISH experiment with oligonucleotides showing (A) dendritic localization (arrowheads) of a particular mRNA in the processes (dendrites) of CA1 pyramidal cells and dentate granule cells as well as in the cell bodies. (B) Distribution of an mRNA confined solely to cell bodies. Exposure times for the two autoradiographs were equal. Images were printed as described in Section 1.8. Olignucleotides, sequences of which were derived from novel rat brain-specific cDNAs identified by a differential screening method, were a kind gift from Dr D. Maréchal and Professor A. Dresse, Department of Pharmacology, University of Liege, Belgium (see Maréchal *et al.*, 1993). DG., dentate granule cells.

information before dipping in emulsion (Wisden *et al.*, 1991a; Tölle *et al.*, 1993). X-ray film resolution is also good enough to provide an indication of mRNA that is present in cell processes such as dendrites (Figure 1.8; see also Garner *et al.*, 1988). X-ray film images, provided that they have been exposed in the linear range, are also easy to quantify by densitometry (see Chapter 7 of this volume).

For X-ray film exposure, slides are stuck to a cardboard sheet (convenient sheets are often supplied as stiffeners in boxes of X-ray film). The slides are attached along the base using autoclave marker tape or a similar type of tape which can easily be peeled off again if the slides are to be dipped in emulsion at some later stage. The cassette must be tight-fitting and must press the film and sections firmly together, otherwise 'out-of-focus' images may result. If this occurs, an extra sheet of cardboard can be added. Cassettes are exposed at room temperature in a vibration-free environment. Mechanical impacts to the

cassette may cause the film to move slightly and a double image will result. If such an accident happens, it is best to develop the film immediately and re-expose. The β-electrons from ^{35}S and ^{33}P are completely absorbed by the film, so exposure at $-70°$C with scintillation screens is not required.

1.5.1 Length of exposure to film

Exposure time depends, of course, on both mRNA abundance and probe specific radio-activity. In our hands, using ^{35}S-labelled probes, exposures vary anywhere between a few days (for some neurofilament-associated protein mRNAs, e.g. MAP-2) and 6 weeks (nicotinic receptor subunit mRNA in rat brain) to obtain a good signal. It is best to carry out a preliminary exposure of 1 week on X-ray film. More often than not, this results in a reasonable image suitable for printing directly on to photographic paper (see Section 1.8). ^{33}P-labelled probes should require, on average, one-third shorter exposure times (see Section 1.3.5).

1.5.2 Types of X-ray film

A detailed consideration of types of X-ray film is given by O'Shea and Gundlach (Chapter 7 of this volume). On a routine basis, including use for publication, we tend to use Kodak XAR-5 film. This film, which is coated with emulsion on both sides, has a grey and slightly grainy base, and can be developed in an automatic Xomat machine. For a slightly higher-resolution image, one can use Kodak SAR-5 film (single-sided emulsion) which, when developed, has a clear blue base. This film must be developed manually. Alternatively some investigators use Amersham Hyperfilm β-max film (high silver content, single sided). Although it requires manual development, it gives faster results than other single-sided films and may be better for low-power photographing on a microscope as it avoids 'double-images' associated with two-sided films at these powers of magnification (Andrew Gundlach, personal communication). All images illustrated in this chapter were made using Kodak

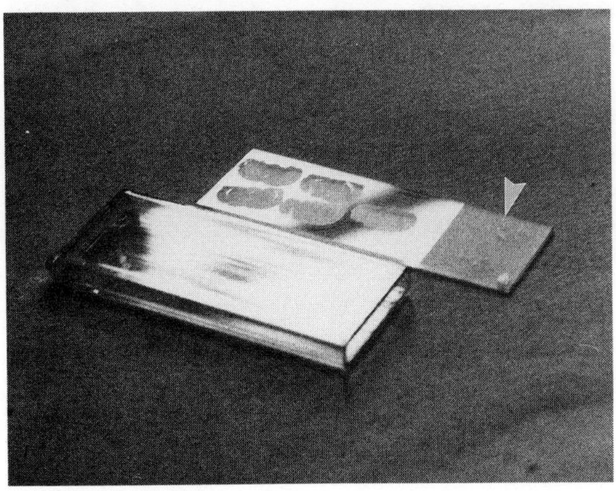

Figure 1.9 A dipping chamber (made by the local glass blower) for coating slides with photographic emulsion. A standard microscope slide (with sections) is shown for scale. Note that one end of the slide (indicated by the arrowhead) is frosted, making it very useful for labelling with pencil.

XAR-5 film and developed in an automatic machine.

1.6 CELLULAR RESOLUTION USING PHOTOGRAPHIC NUCLEAR EMULSION

Note that aspects of nuclear emulsion studies are also discussed by O'Shea and Gundlach in Chapter 7. The use of emulsion for double-labelling studies employing alkaline phosphatase-labelled and ^{35}S-labelled oligonucleotides is described by Augood *et al.* in Chapter 8.

In order to achieve detailed cellular resolution, which is essential for very small organisms such as insects and some vertebrate embryos, sections have to be dipped in photographic nuclear emulsion. For example, on the basis of X-ray film autoradiographs alone, it is not possible to determine whether the GABA$_A$ receptor γ1 subunit mRNA is in Purkinje cells or Bergmann glial cells, as both types of cell body are colocalized in the cerebellum (Figure 1.10). Other examples of emulsion-generated autoradiographs are shown in Figure 5.3, Figure 6.1, Figure 7.4 and Figures 8.7 and 8.8.

The combined method for dipping hybridized

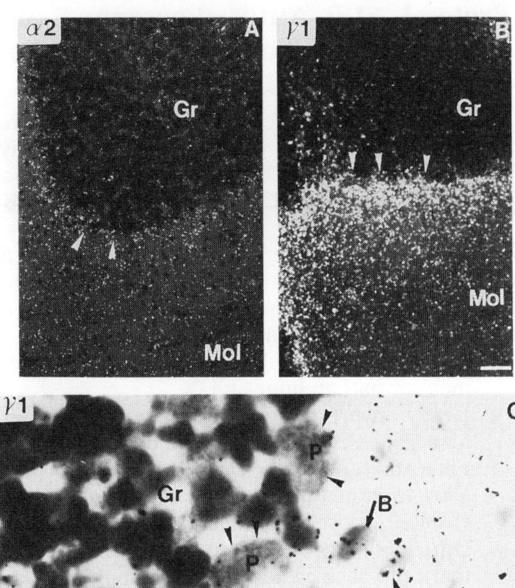

Figure 1.10 Detection of mRNA encoding the γ1 subunit of GABA$_A$ receptors in putative Bermann glia of the rat cerebellum using emulsion autoradiography. The α2 subunit and γ1 subunit probes hybridize only to the Purkinje cell layer as assessed from X-ray film autoradiographic images (see Laurie *et al.*, 1992). The α2 signal is very weak. Examination of the origins of this signal with photographic emulsion confirm that the signal results from hybridization to the Purkinje cell layer (arrowheads). The α2 signal is a halo of silver grains under darkfield optics, along the border between the granule (Gr) and molecular cell layers (Mol), the granule cells themselves being unlabelled (A). For the γ1 subunit mRNA, a dense cluster of silver grains originates at the granule cell/molecular layer border (arrowheads) and extends out into the molecular level (B). High-power brightfield optics using a 100 × lens with immersion oil reveals that the Purkinje cells (designated P, black arrowheads) themselves are unlabelled by the γ1 probe (C). Silver grains are clustered over small cells (designated B, arrows) surrounding the Purkinje cells, with the granule cells being unlabelled. The position of these labelled cells suggests that they may be Bergmann glia. Photomicrographs were obtained with a Zeiss Axioplan microscope. Reproduced from Laurie *et al.* (1992).

sections in photographic emulsion, and subsequent exposure, developing and thionin staining is given in Protocol 1.9. When dipping sections, it is a good idea to include a few blank slides as a

Protocol 1.9 Autoradiography of sections using photographic emulsion.

1. The emulsion is mixed on the day of use. All procedures are performed under safe-lighting using Kodak 6B or equivalent filters. Prewarm 25 ml of water/0.5% glycerol in a 50 ml polypropylene screw-top Falcon tube to 43°C. The entire procedure is performed in a water bath.
2. Add solid emulsion shreds[a] to the prewarmed water/glycerol so that it displaces the liquid to the 50 ml mark. This makes a 1:1 ratio of emulsion water. The emulsion can best be scraped out of its stock bottle using wooden cocktail sticks.
3. Wrap the Falcon tube in aluminium foil and allow the emulsion to melt for half an hour at 43°C.
4. *Gently* invert the mixture several times in order to produce a homogeneous solution. Avoid creating bubbles.
5. Filter mixture through muslin cloth into the dipping chamber[b] and allow to stand for several minutes to remove air bubbles. The dipping chamber is also maintained at 43°C.
6. Dip slides individually into the chamber, allow to drain and then place to dry in a rack over a humid environment (damp tissue paper). Slides are allowed to dry in complete darkness for 2–3 h.
7. Transfer slides to light-tight slide boxes, e.g. BDH/Merck 'staining rack' and 'troughs'. These are black polyacetate boxes with push-fit lids (size 100 × 85 × 55 mm) each containing a sachet of silica gel. Seal boxes with insulation tape. Store at 4°C for the required time (usually between 4 and 8 weeks). In our experience, the inclusion of fresh silica gel is important, as, if damp emulsion-coated slides are left for long periods, moulds tend to grow over the sections. Remarkably, the moulds can digest away most of the section.
8. On the day of development, slide boxes are allowed to warm up to room temperature. This prevents moisture condensing on them and possibly interfering with the emulsion. Under safe-light conditions (Kodak 6B), slides are transferred into glass racks.
9. Immerse slides in 250 ml of D19 developer[c] (17°C) for 2 min[d]. After developing, immerse slides in deionized water for 30 s.
10. Transfer slides into 250 ml of a freshly prepared solution of 30% sodium thiosulphate for 2 min. You can also use Ilford Pan paper fixer (200 ml of pan fixer/litre).
11. Transfer slides into 250 ml of distilled water for 2 min. Normal lights can be turned on at this point.
12. Wash in distilled water twice for 10 min.
13. Allow slides to air-dry for half an hour.
14. Sections are now ready to be stained[e]. Immerse sections in a 0.1% solution of thionin for several minutes[f].
15. Transfer sections into 70% ethanol to remove as much of the stain as required. Transfer sections into 95% ethanol for several minutes. Transfer sections into 100% ethanol for several minutes. Transfer sections into Histoclear (National Diagnostics) for several minutes.
16. Drain the sections of Histoclear and mount with glass coverslips and DPX mounting medium (BDH/Merck).

---

[a] Emulsion is Ilford K5 stored at 4°C. We prefer the K5 emulsion to the commonly used Kodak NTB2 emulsion, because the Ilford brand requires no aliquoting before use. Kodak NTB2 is discussed in Section 5.4.2, p. 53.

[b] The dipping chamber is a glass vessel about the same depth as the microscope slides (see Figure 1.9). It is best to get these made by your local glass blower.

[c] D19 developer (Kodak) is made up from the powder exactly according to the suppliers' instructions. It is stored in light-tight (dark glass) bottles at room

temperature. When dissolved, D19 is a pale-straw colour. If it is excessively discoloured (dark brown), make up a fresh stock.

[d] Developer is cooled to 17°C on ice.

[e] Dr Andrew Gundlach has pointed out to us a method popularized by the Hokfelt group in Sweden. This is simply to photograph developed emulsions under water or glycerol coverslip with no counterstain. This helps identify fibre tracts and grey matter regions when viewed under darkfield. If desired, sections can then be rephotographed following Nissl staining. This works well for regions such as the medulla oblongata and nucleus of the solitary tract.

[f] Thionin/Lauth's Violet, acetate salt (Sigma, No T-3387) is dissolved in 0.1 M acetic acid, 0.1 M sodium acetate to make a 1% (w/v) stock solution. This stock solution is diluted tenfold in 0.1 M acetic acid, 0.1 M sodium acetate to make a 0.1% working solution. Filter through cotton wool before use; this removes any large particles of undissolved dye which could precipitate on to the sections.

control for emulsion background. These blank slides can be placed in a separate box and should be developed the day after the dipping – there should be very little background. If something has gone wrong – the worst scenario being that they are completely fogged – it may be that the emulsion was exposed to light at some point. However, it may still be possible to rescue the sections! Shughrue and Dorsa (1992) report that after accidental exposure to light, the emulsion can be melted off the slides as follows. Slides with fogged emulsion are placed in 1 × SSC at 55°C for 5 min to melt the emulsion off. They are then placed in 1 × SSC at 42°C for 3 min and then at room temperature in 0.1 × SSC for 5 min. The slides are then fixed at room temperature in Kodak fixer, rinsed for 5 min in 0.1 × SSC and dehydrated through a graded series of ethanols and air-dried. The slides can then be redipped.

Coating slides with photographic emulsion appears to be less sensitive than exposure to X-ray film. With ^{35}S-labelled probes, it is a general 'rule of thumb' that exposure of slides dipped in emulsion requires *five times longer* than exposure of the same section to X-ray film. Specifically, a 1-week exposure to X-ray film requires 5 weeks with dipped emulsion. In practice, we usually expose dipped sections for a minimum of 8–12 weeks to generate *strong* clustering of silver grains over cell bodies. Emulsion studies can be quantified by counting silver grains (Chapter 7). The use of chemically modified oligonucleotides and deoxygenin-labelled cRNA probes (see Chapters 8, 9 and 10 for non-radioactive ISH) promises to eliminate the need to use emulsion for qualitative studies, and the associated long delays before one can see the result (or lack thereof!).

1.7 PHILOSOPHY OF CONTROLS FOR ISH

Tissue sections contain many surfaces and sites which can trap probes and thus generate misleading results. As discussed in detail by Uhl (1987), there are no completely satisfactory universal controls for ISH studies. In our opinion, for ISH using oligonucleotides, the two best controls are competition hybridizations with excess concentrations of unlabelled oligonucleotides and the reproduction of identical autoradiographic patterns with several (i.e. at least two) independent oligonucleotides built to hybridize to different parts of the mRNA. These two types of control are illustrated in Figure 1.11. As assessed by ISH on a horizontal rat brain section with a ^{35}S-labelled 45-mer (KA-2a), the mRNA encoding a subunit of a high-affinity kainate excitatory amino acid receptor termed KA-2 is found to be abundantly expressed in many parts of the rat brain, e.g. neocortex, hippocampus and granule cell layer of the cerebellum (Figure 1.11a; Herb *et al.*, 1992). When a parallel horizontal section is hybridized with buffer containing both the same unlabelled and radiolabelled probe, most of the signal is competed out (Figure 1.11b; see also Figure 2.3). Some pattern lines remain over the meninges (the ventricle lining of the brain), and this is therefore interpreted to be non-specific (arrowheads in Figures 1.11a and 1.11b). The principle behind

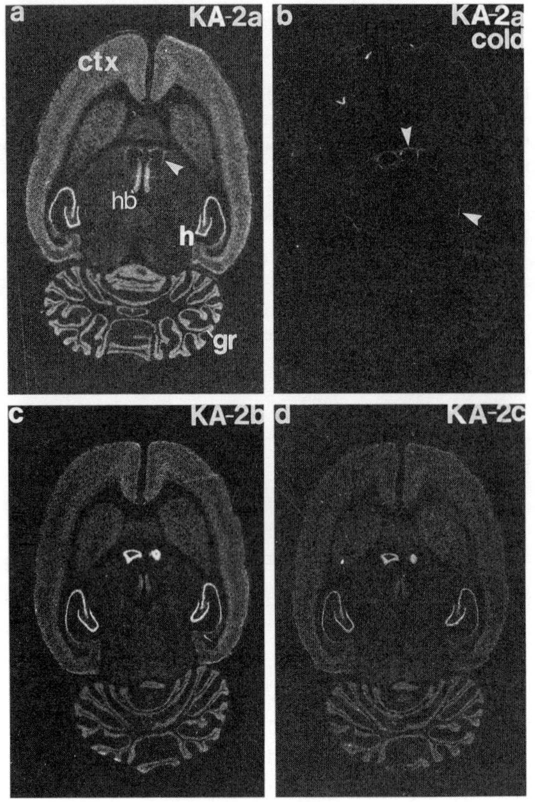

Figure 1.11 Controls for ISH. X-ray film autoradiographic image in (a) resulted from hybridization of a ^{35}S-labelled KA-2a oligonucleotide to a horizontal rat brain section. The image in (b) was a parallel hybridization, the hybridization buffer of which contained a 100-fold excess of unlabelled KA-2a in addition to the ^{35}S-labelled KA-2a, everything else being identical. The arrowheads indicate that some non-specific hybridization is present over the ventricle linings (meninges). Images in (c) and (d) are hybridizations performed with oligonucleotides KA-2b and KA-2c, which hybridize to different regions of the KA-2 mRNA (see Herb *et al.*, 1992). ctx, neocortex; h, hippocampus; hb, medial habenulae; gr, cerebellar granule cells.

this competition control is that specific binding is saturable (i.e. of finite amount), whereas non-specific binding increases linearly, and, within the range of probe concentrations used in these experiments, can be regarded as 'infinite'. See Protocol 1.5, footnote *a* for experimental details of setting up the competition hybridization. Figures 1.11c and 1.11d are autoradiographs obtained from two further distinct 40- and

45-mer oligonucleotides (KA-2b and KA-2c, designed to hybridize to different regions of the KA-2 mRNA). The pattern is essentially the same as that obtained with the original KA-2 probe, thus confirming specificity.

There are other controls which are less informative for the *exact* specificity of a particular probe, but which may be useful when setting up the system for the very first time.

(i)   Hybridization with a labelled sense (coding-strand) oligonucleotide with the same length, base composition and specific activity as the antisense probe. An absence of a signal with such a sense probe does *not* guarantee that the signal obtained with the antisense probe is specific. The antisense probe could still be cross-hybridizing to a related sequence. However, the sense probe is a useful control for determining general parameters of non-specific hybridization to the section.

(ii) Pretreatment of the sections before hybridization with RNAse A invariably destroys the signal. This control is performed by removing sections from ethanol storage and air-drying. They are then transferred to a continental trough containing 250 ml of $2 \times$ SSC with 20 µg ml^{-1} RNAse A (see Sambrook *et al.* (1989) for preparation of RNAse A stocks and Blumberg (1987) for the safe handling of RNAse A). Sections are incubated at 37°C for half an hour. They are then dehydrated through $0.1 \times$ SSC, 70% and 95% ethanol and hybridized with labelled probe in the standard manner (Protocol 1.5). It is important to keep glassware and solutions that come into contact with RNAse A separate from that used for the main experiments.

(iii) Northern blots. If a probe, used at appropriate stringency, gives a particular auto-radiographic pattern after hybridization to brain sections, it invariably hybridizes to discrete band(s) on a Northern blot, given that enough mRNA has been loaded and hybridization and washing conditions resemble the ISH experiment. This is frequently cited as a confirmation of probe specificity for ISH. However, this really only

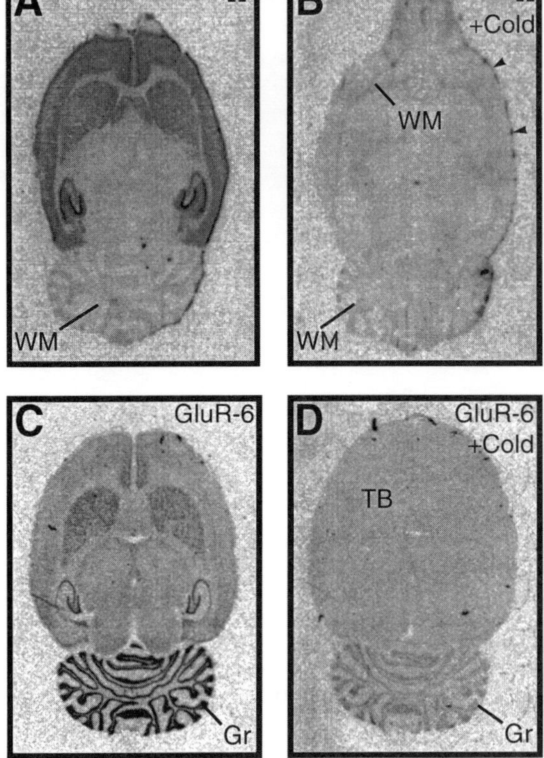

Figure 1.12 (A) and (B) show the result of hybridizing an oligonucleotide targeting an mRNA (Ω) which is found only in the forebrain. This was a 'bad' experiment, because for some reason, the white matter (WM) bound the probe non-specifically. This can clearly be seen in (B), as judged from hybridization with a 100-fold excess of unlabelled (cold) oligonucleotide, where the white matter labelling is the same intensity as in the experiment of (A). The arrowheads in (B) indicate an artefact where the edge of the section has trapped probe. Some probes can bind non-specifically to the cerebellar granule cells (Gr), especially if their poly($[^{35}S]$A) tail is too long. This is illustrated in (C) (radiolabelled probe only) and (D) (radiolabelled probe and 100-fold excess of cold probe) using an oligonucleotide that hybridizes to the GluR-6 mRNA of high-affinity kainate receptors. (D) also illustrates the general section background (TB) as determined by hybridization with excess probe. All images were for the same exposure time on to X-ray film. Note that in contrast with the other Figures in this chapter, which were made manually by hand-printing on to photographic paper, this Figure was produced by digitizing the X-ray film image on an Optotech Scanner and processing it on an Adobe Photoshop program with an Apple Macintosh computer. The digitized image was then printed directly out on a Canon CLC 300 photocopier.

demonstrates specificity if *different* oligonucleotides, recognizing *different* parts of the mRNA hybridize to the *same* band(s). Northern blots may provide a useful confirmation of the ISH result if mRNA abundance from dissected tissues is shown to reflect the autoradiographic distribution. However, in our opinion, if it is not necessary to know mRNA size, ISH with multiple probes is adequate (assuming there to be no alternative splicing). Northern blots may be an important control if one is not sure about the stringency of hybridization used in the ISH experiment.

If the conditions for ISH on brain are followed *exactly* as presented in this chapter, particularly with regard to probe concentrations, non-specific signals are usually virtually absent from vertebrate brain and embryonic sections.

1.7.1 Artefacts

In spite of everything, various artefacts are occasionally produced! For example, Figures 1.12A and 1.12B show the result of hybridizing an oligonucleotide targeting an mRNA found only in the forebrain. This was a 'bad' experiment, because for some unknown reason, the white matter bound the probe non-specifically. This can clearly be seen in Figure 1.12B, as judged from hybridization with a 100-fold excess of unlabelled (cold) oligonucleotide. The labelling of the white matter is at the same intensity as in the experiment of Figure 1.12A. The cause of this labelling is not clear, with only a very small number (a few percent) of individual brains giving such backgrounds. Delipidation with chloroform before hybridization may help (see Protocol 1.10), although storage in absolute ethanol is usually sufficient. Similarly, we occasionally produce sections in which probes bind non-specifically to the granule cells of rodent cerebellum (illustrated in Figures 1.12C and 1.12D) when a probe that hybridizes to a glutamate receptor subunit mRNA, GluR-6, is used. This is usually due to the poly ($[^{35}S]$A) tail being too long, i.e. counts greater than 400 000 d.p.m. μl^{-1} of labelled probe.

Protocol 1.10 Optional pretreatment of sections before hybridization[a]

For all the steps listed below, use clean glassware and sterile water to make up all solutions. Use 250 ml of each solution in BDH/Merck glass staining troughs (see Figure 1.2).
1. Transfer sections straight from 95% ethanol storage into 1 × PBS.
2. Transfer into 0.25% (v/v) acetic anhydride in 0.1 M triethanolamine/ HCl, pH 8.0/0.9% NaCl for 10 min at room temperature[b].
3. Transfer into 70% ethanol for 1 min.
4. Transfer into 95% ethanol for 2 min.
5. Transfer into 100% ethanol for 1 min.
6. Transfer into 100% chloroform for 5 min.
7. Transfer back through 100% (1 min) and 95% (1 min) ethanol.
8. Air-dry sections and proceed to Protocol 1.5, step 1.

[a] This protocol is taken from Young *et al.* (1986a) and may be beneficial for tissues that give high non-specific binding.
[b] To prepare the acetic anhydride solution, add 3.3 ml of triethanolamine (it comes as a viscous liquid), 1.25 g of NaCl and 1.0 ml of conc. HCl per 250 ml of sterile water. Mix well. Just before use, add 625 µl of acetic anhydride. Stir well with a sterile pipette tip.

1.8 PRINTING AND PRESENTATION OF AUTORADIOGRAPHS FOR PUBLICATION

Although this 'non-scientific' section may be obvious to some readers, many with no prior experience of histology or darkroom expertise might appreciate a discussion of useful ways of producing photographic images of ISH auto-radiographs for the purposes of publication. Along with cutting high-quality sections, the preparation of a histology plate is the part of the whole ISH procedure that requires the most finesse and judgement.

Production of the image is very straightforward. After exposure and development, it is wise to cut the sheets of X-ray film into strips and store them in the type of plastic wallets used for protecting developed 35 mm films against scratching. Such strips of X-ray film can be inserted directly into a photographic enlarger (just as for normal negatives), and a reverse image can be printed on to photographic paper. This results in a pseudo-'darkfield' image, with black areas of signal on X-ray film appearing white on the printed paper. Choice of paper grade can be critical in presenting an image. It is generally best to use a high-contrast paper type. We recommend Agfa grade-6 Rapidoprint line paper (TP6 WPt2).

Printing an autoradiograph which will be used for publication with the correct amount of contrast is to some extent subjective. One should, of course, try to match the printed image to that on the X-ray film in terms of intensity of signal. However, to a naive observer with no knowledge of the signal intensity on the film, the distribution of mRNA can be made to change rather vividly depending on printing conditions. Figure 1.13 illustrates this effect. The same X-ray film autoradiograph (that of AMPA/kainate receptor GluR-A subunit mRNA in the rat brain) was used to produce all four pictures. However, exposure time in the enlarger varied by 5 s increments. All images were developed and fixed for equal times (Ilford Pan developer, diluted 1:9, 30 s, Ilford Pan fixer, diluted 1:3, 5 min). Image A (Figure 1.13) is definitely underexposed ('underprinted') with the mRNA appearing to be abundant everywhere. However, without knowledge of the primary autoradiograph, it is not clear whether B, C or D represents the 'correct' distribution (Figure 1.13). It is in fact image B. Image D is extreme and is 'overprinted' with the GluR-A gene apparently expressed

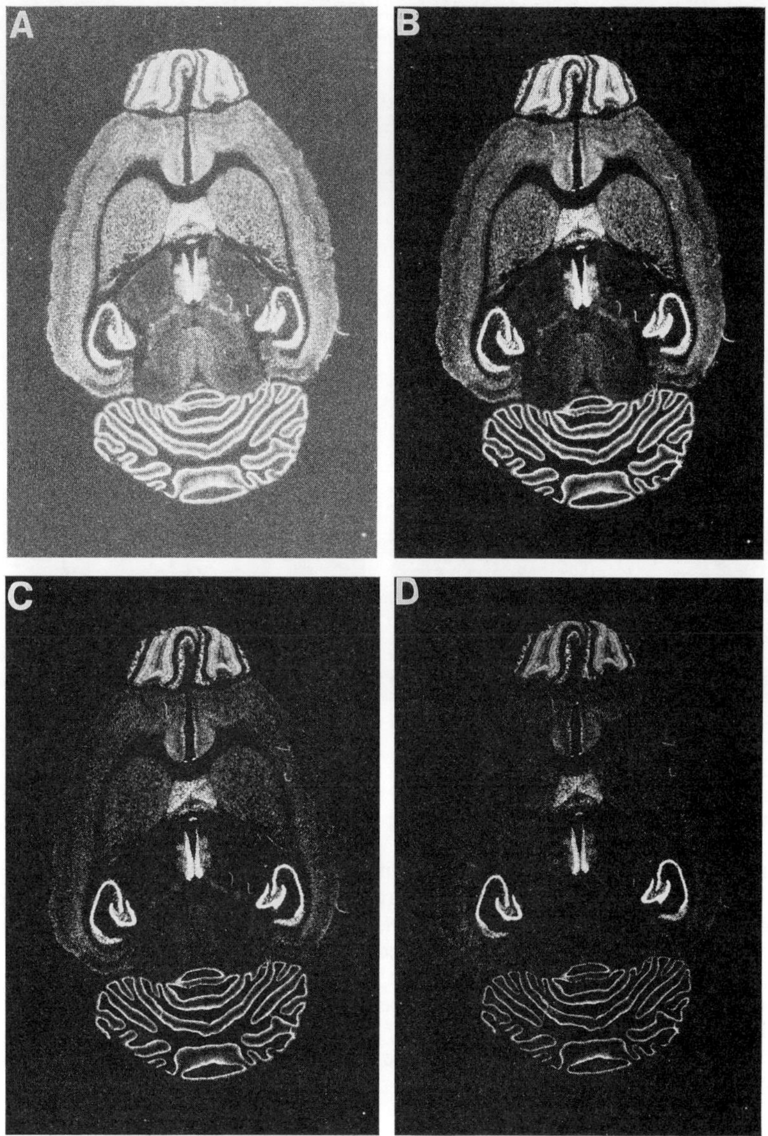

Figure 1.13 Printing X-ray film autoradiographs. The same image of the AMPA-kainate receptor GluR-A subunit mRNA distribution in a rat brain horizontal section (Keinänen *et al.*, 1990) has been printed in all four photographs, but exposure time of light to the photographic paper (Agfa grade 6) differed by 5 s increments. (A) 10 s; (B) 15 s, (C) 20 s and (D) 25 s. All prints were developed for the same length of time (30 s in Ilford Pan paper developer) and fixed for 5 min in Ilford Pan fix. The oligonucleotide specific for the GluR-A subunit mRNA was as detailed in Keinänen *et al.* (1990).

mainly in the hippocampus and habenulae, with very little neocortical expression. It is as well to be aware of these possibilities when examining published autoradiographs.

It is often desirable to match an X-ray film image with its corresponding Nissl stained section; a convenient and rapid alternative to taking a picture of the whole section on a low-powered microscope is to simply insert the stained slide directly into the enlarger. The appropriate section is stained with thionin using the method given in Protocol 1.9, steps 13–16, and mounted under a coverslip. After the slide has dried, dust particles are cleaned off by wiping

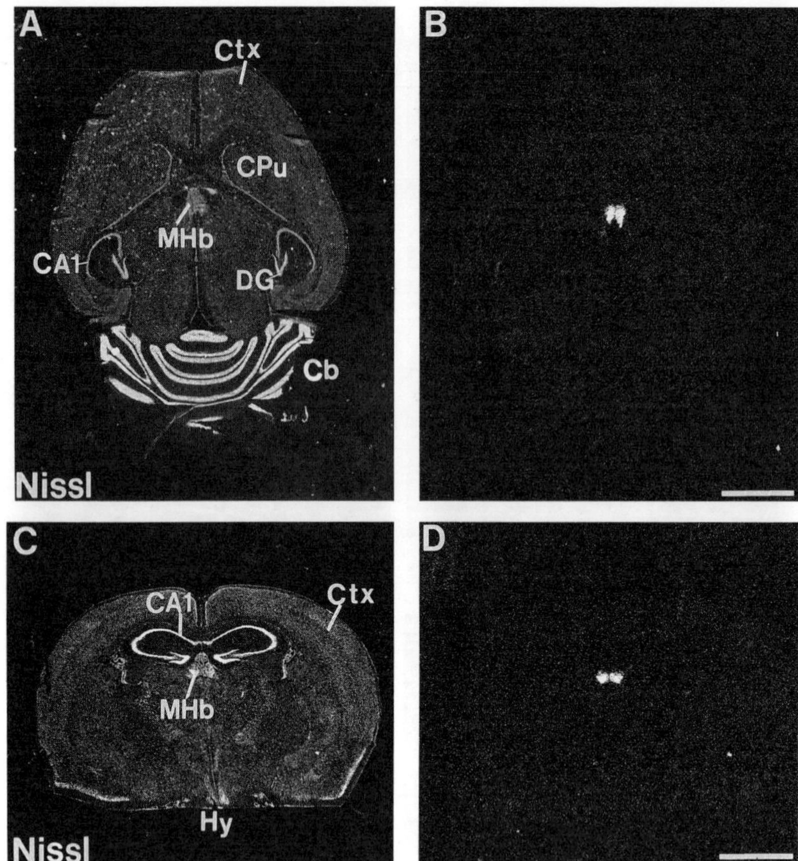

Figure 1.14 Printing Nissl stains of sections. X-ray film autoradiographs (B and D) were produced using an oligonucleotide targeting an mRNA encoding the serotonin 5B receptor that is found to be largely restricted to the medial habenulae in adult mice (Matthes *et al.*, 1993; W. Wisden and M. Voigt, unpublished). After exposure to the X-ray film, the sections were stained with thionin (Protocol 1.9) and the microscope slides were printed directly in the enlarger (A and C), at the same magnification as used for the X-ray film, to generate an image of the entire section. It can be seen that areas of high cell density which appear white on the photographic paper, such as the granule layer of the cerebellum and dentate gyrus of the hippocampus, are devoid of signal. Cb. cerebellum; CPu, caudate-putamen; Ctx, neocortex; DG, dentate granule cells; Hy, hypothalamus; MHb, medial habenulae

with 70% ethanol. The X-ray film image is first printed, and then the slide is inserted into the enlarger and printed at exactly the same magnification as used for the X-ray film. The resulting image will have regions of white corresponding to the blue Nissl stain (Figure 1.14). This printing technique also gives very nice results for vertebrate embryo sections (see Figure 2.1). Printing the Nissl stain may require a different exposure time in the enlarger from that used to print the X-ray film.

Advances in desktop publishing mean that digitized images may be the future routine way of presenting ISH autoradiographs. For example, Figure 1.12 was generated by scanning the X-ray film autoradiographs with an Optotech scanner which inputted directly into an Apple Macintosh computer running on Cirrus software. An Adobe Photoshop desktop publishing program (again on the Macintosh) was used to manipulate all the features of the image on the computer screen (e.g. contrast, brightness and lettering). The final version was printed out on a Canon CLC 300 colour photocopier. This is altogether a much quicker and neater process than printing pictures with an enlarger, cutting the images to size, assembling them into a plate, Letrasetting them and finally rephotographing them to make copies of the finished Figure. The electronic method will save weeks of work if large numbers of autoradiographs are to be assembled into Plates. However, if Figure 1.13 illustrated ways of manipulating data by hand printing, then the possibilities with digitized images are even greater! Using this method, different tissue and film backgrounds can be normalized and made to appear equal, although one useful feature is that obvious distracting artefacts such as scratches and blotches are easy to remove. Thus, authors of papers should always state how the figures were produced.

ACKNOWLEDGEMENTS

We gratefully acknowledge the support of the Wellcome Trust (to BJM) and the Medical Research Council UK (to BJM and WW). WW thanks Professor Peter H. Seeburg (ZMBH, University of Heidelberg) for advice and practical input, particularly with regard to probe labelling. We are very appreciative of the outstanding technical support of Ulla Keller (ZMBH, University of Heidelberg) who performed many of the experiments illustrated in this chapter. Thanks also to Drs David J. Laurie (ZMBH, University of Heidelberg) and Andrew Gundlach (University of Melbourne, Australia) for critically reading the manuscript and providing useful suggestions. Stuart Ingham (Visual Aids Department, MRC Centre, Cambridge, UK) kindly generated Figure 1.12 and explained the digitizing system.

REFERENCES

Albretsen, C., Haukanes, B.I., Aasland, R. & Kleppe, K. (1988) *Anal. Biochem.* **170**, 193–202.

Barton, A.J.L., Pearson, R.C.A., Najlerahim, A. & Harrison, P.J. (1993) *J. Neurochem.* **61**, 1–11.

Blumberg, D.D. (1987) *Methods Enzymol.* **152**, 20–24.

Dagerlind, A., Friberg, K., Bean, A.J. & Hökfelt, T. (1992) *Histochemistry* **98**, 39–49

Du Pont Biotech Update (1992) **7(1)**, p. 12.

Erlander, M.G., Lovenberg, T.W., Baron, B.M., De Lecea, L., Danielson, P.E., Racke, M., Slone, A.L., Siegel, B.W., Foye, P.E., Cannon, K.,

Burns, J.E. & Sutcliffe, J.G. (1993) *Proc. Natl. Acad. Sci. USA* **90**, 3452–3456.

Eschenfeldt, W.H., Puskas, R.S. & Berger, S.L. (1987) *Methods Enzymol.* **152**, 337–342.

Garner, G.C., Tucker, R.P. & Matus, A. (1988) *Nature* **336**, 674–677

Herb, A., Burnashev, N., Werner, P., Sakmann, B., Wisden, W. & Seeburg, P.H. (1992) *Neuron* **8**, 775–785.

Keinänen, K., Wisden, W., Sommer, B., Werner, P., Herb, A., Verdoorn, T.A., Sakmann, B. & Seeburg, P.H. (1990) *Science* **249**, 556–560

Lathe, R. (1985) *J. Mol. Biol.* **183**, 1–12.

Laurie, D.J., Seeburg, P.H. & Wisden, W. (1992) *J. Neurosci.* **12**, 1063–1076.

Lewis, M.E., Sherman, T.G. & Watson, S.J. (1985). *Peptides* **6 (Suppl. 2)**, 75–87.

Lewis, M.E., Krause, R.G. & Roberts-Lewis, J.M. (1988) *Synapse,* **2**, 308–316.

Lomeli, H., Sprengel, R., Laurie, D.J., Köhr, G., Herb, A., Seeburg, P.H. & Wisden, W. (1993) *FEBS Lett.* **315**, 318–322.

Maréchal, D., Forceille, C., Breyer, D., Delapierre, D. & Dresse, A. (1993) *Anal. Biochem.* **208**, 330–333.

Matthes, H., Boschert, U., Amlaiky, N., Grailhe, R., Plassat, J-L., Muscatelli, F., Mattei, M-G. & Hen, R. (1993) *Mol. Pharmacol.* **43**, 313–319.

Noguchi, K., Kowalski, R., Traub, R., Solodkin, A., Iadarola, M.J. & Ruda, M.A. (1991) *Mol. Brain Res.* **10**, 227–233.

Pittius, C.W., Kley, N., Loeffler, J.P. & Hoellt, V. (1985) *EMBO J.* **4**, 1257–1260.

Persohn, E., Melherbe, P. & Richards, J.G. (1992) *J. Comp. Neurol.* **326**, 193–216.

Rattray, M. & Priestley, J.V. (1993) *Amersham Life Science News Letter*, issue **11**, p. 4.

Ross, B.M., Knowler, J.T. & McCulloch, J. (1992) *J. Neurochem.* **58**, 1810–1819.

Sambrook, J., Fritsch, E.F. & Maniatis, T. (1989) *Molecular cloning: a laboratory manual*, 2nd edn. Cold Spring Harbor Laboratory Press, Cold Spring Harbor, NY

Shughrue, P.J. & Dorsa, D.M. (1992) *BioTechniques* **13**, 498–499.

Singer, M. & Berg, P. (1992) *Genes and genomes.* University Science Books, Blackwell, pp. 258–260.

Sommer, B., Kainänen, K., Verdoorn, T.A., Wisden, W., Burnashev, N., Herb, A., Köhler, M., Takagi, T., Sakmann, B. & Seeburg, P.H. (1990) *Science* **249**, 1580–1585.

Tölle, T.R., Berthele, A., Zieglgänsberger, W., Seeburg, P.H. & Wisden, W. (1993) *J. Neurosci.* (in press).

Uhl, G.R. (ed.) (1987) *In situ hybridization in brain.* Plenum Press, New York.

Uhl, G.R., Cwickel, B., Pagnonis, C. & Habener, J. (1985) *Ann. Neurol.* **18**, 149.

Wahl, G.M., Berger, S.L. & Kimmel, A.R. (1987) *Methods Enzymol.* **152**, 399–407.

Wisden, W., Errington, M.L., Williams, S., Dunnett, S.B., Waters, C., Hitchcock, D., Evan, G., Bliss, T.V.P. & Hunt, S.P. (1990) *Neuron* **4**, 603.

Wisden, W., Gundlach, A.L., Barnard, E.A., Seeburg, P.H. & Hunt, S.P. (1991a) *Mol. Brain Res.* **10**, 179–183.

Wisden, W., Morris, B.J. & Hunt, S.P. (1991b) In *Molecular neurobiology: a practical approach.* J. Chad and H. Wheal (eds). IRL Press/Oxford University Press, Oxford, pp. 205–225.

Young, W.S. III (1989) *Methods Enzymol.* **168**, 702–709.

Young, W.S. III, Mezey, E. & Siegel, R.E. (1986a) *Neurosci. Lett.* **70**, 198–203.

Young, W.S. III, Bonner, T.I. & Brann, M.R. (1986b) *Proc. Natl. Acad. Sci. USA* **83**, 9827

Zagursky, R., Conway, P.S. & Kashdan, M.A. (1991) *Biotechniques* **11**, 36–38

Processing vertebrate embryonic and early postnatal tissue for *in situ* hybridization

DAVID J. LAURIE* & PETRA C.U. SCHROTZ†

* Centre for Molecular Biology (ZMBH), and † Institute for Neurobiology, Im Neuenheimer Feld 282* and 364†, University of Heidelberg, Heidelberg, D-69120 Germany

2.1 INTRODUCTION

The analysis of gene expression by *in situ* hybridization during development of the central nervous system is increasingly important for a variety of biological fields. Determination of the onset of expression of a gene in early embryonic stages, and of changes in its temporal and spatial expression during development can give valuable information about its potential role or function, especially with regard to involvement in cellular proliferation, migration and differentiation. Reliable and presentable data require good-quality sections from accurately aged animals (Figure 2.1). Patience and care are therefore necessary to dissect, manipulate and prepare the delicate tissues from these stages without damage or distortion. This chapter describes steps and hints useful for preparing embryonic and early postnatal (P0–P20) tissue for the *in situ* protocol outlined in Chapter 1. These methods have been used by us to study the developmental expression profiles of mRNAs for γ-aminobutyric acid (GABA$_A$) and N-methyl-D-aspartate (NMDA) receptor subunits (Laurie *et al.*, 1992; H. Monyer *et al.*, unpublished) and cytoskeletal proteins (P.C.U. Schrotz & W.B. Huttner, unpublished).

2.2 STANDARDIZING ANIMAL AGE

Mouse and rat are useful species as they have a short gestation period (20–21 days). The embryonic ages described in this chapter are those for the mouse. Approximately equivalent stages of rat development are given in Table 2.1.

2.2.1 Embryos

In order to obtain precisely staged embryos, the mating period should be as short as possible and only females with a definite postcoital vaginal plug should be used. See Theiler (1989) or Rugh

IN SITU HYBRIDIZATION PROTOCOLS FOR THE BRAIN
ISBN 0–12–759919–3

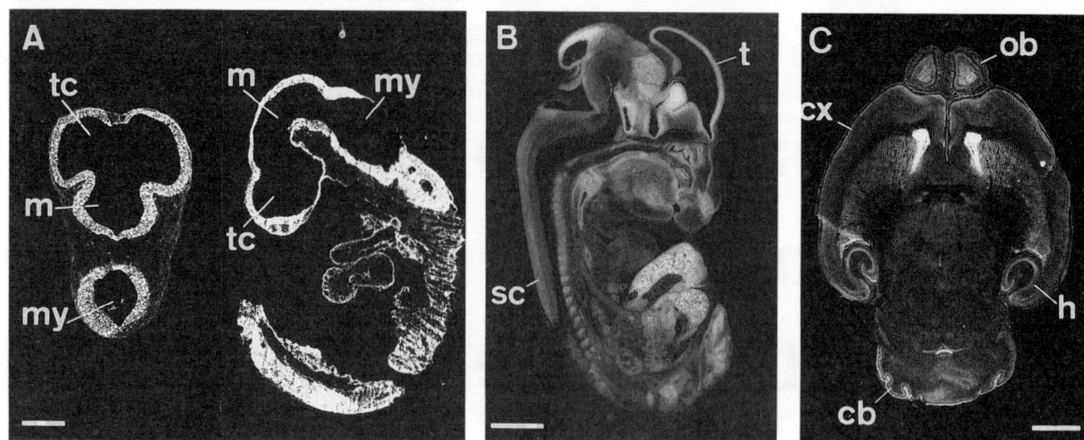

Figure 2.1 Nissl-stained sections. (A) Prefixed mouse E9.5 embryos in transverse (left) and parasagittal (right) sections, (B) E14 rat embryo (sagittal), and (C) rat P0 postnatal brain (horizontal). Abbreviations: cb, cerebellum; cx, cortex; h, hippocampus; m, mesecoele; my, myelocoele; ob, olfactory bulb; sc, spinal cord; t, telencephalon; tc, telocoele. Bars = 0.5 mm (A) and 2 mm (B and C).

Table 2.1 An approximate correlation between mouse and rat embryonic development. Compiled from data by Goedbloed & Smits-van Prooije (1986), Theiler (1989), Rugh (1991) and Kaufman (1992).

Approximate number of somites	Stage of embryonic development (gestational age in days)	
	Mouse	Rat
1–7	8	9
8–12	8.5	9.8
13–21	9	10.5
22–26	9.5	11.2
27–33	10	12
34–38	10.5	12.5
39–43	11	13

(1991) for more details. For greatest efficiency, matings should be set up in the early morning (e.g. about 8 a.m.) for a period of 1 h. Since oestrus normally begins around midnight, morning matings have the advantage that all the receptive eggs are already present in the oviduct and can be fertilized immediately and approximately simultaneously. Such matings reduce aging errors of embryos to under 2 h. The vaginal plug is visible for only a few hours and from the point of its detection we assign the age of embryonic day 0 (E0). With evening matings, the spermatozoa must survive in the female reproductive tract until the following ovulation, when ova are ready for fertilization in a sequential manner. Long overnight matings can therefore result in an age range of up to 16 h, with resultant embryos being at different stages of development (Juurlink & Federoff, 1980).

If a more exact staging of development is required, individual embryonic ages can be confirmed by:

(i) examination of the somites (Rugh, 1991)
(ii) examination of paw, eye or ear development (Rugh, 1991)
(iii) measurement of crown–rump length (Dunnett & Björklund, 1992)

In addition, E8 and E9 embryos can be distinguished by posture; an E8 embryo is dorsally curved, whereas at E9 the tail faces the ventral surface of the head (Theiler, 1989; Kaufman, 1992).

2.2.2 Postnatal animals

For postnatal brains the first 24 h after birth is termed by us postnatal day 0 (P0), following the reasons outlined in Paxinos *et al.* (1991).

2.3 EXCISION OF TISSUE

2.3.1 Embryo

A brief description of uterine dissection procedures and embryo excision will be given. More detail can be found in Hogan *et al.* (1986) and Dunnett & Björklund (1992). Pregnant females are killed by cervical dislocation and the uteri dissected out from the abdomen, rinsed in ice-cold buffer (200 mM HEPES, pH 7.4, in diethyl pyrocarbonate (DEPC)-treated water) and placed in a second Petri dish of the same buffer. During dissection the buffer must be kept cold. We recommend HEPES buffer rather than phosphate-buffered saline as it keeps the tissue mass in a better condition, especially during long preparation times. The HEPES buffer ideally should be fresh but can be stored at 4°C for up to 4 days.

For early (E8–E10) embryos there are several degrees of preparation:

2.3.1.1 Uterus

The fastest and simplest method is to leave the embryos *in utero*. The uterus is cut into segments of 1–3 decidua each which are arranged on a strip of aluminium foil. The foil is placed on dry ice until the tissue is completely frozen (approx. 5 min). This method is useful for E10 embryos, but tissue morphology is not ideally preserved.

2.3.1.2 Deciduum

The excised uterus can be partitioned into a vascularized dorsal face and a ventral face where the early E8–E10 embryo is located and easily accessible. Using a dissecting microscope, the decidua (egg-shaped structures inside the thick muscular myometrium) are dissected out by sliding very fine forceps (Dumont no. 5) between the muscle layer and the deciduum on the dorsal side and peeling away the myometrium. Care must be taken not to harm the pressurized deciduum as it may rupture, causing the embryo to be expelled and damaged. Especially at these early stages when the tissue integrity is still quite loose, it is advisable to fix the whole deciduum or the completely excised embryo. The deciduum is transferred into fixative with a small spatula (Section 2.3.1.4) or the embryo is isolated (Section 2.3.1.3).

2.3.1.3 Embryo

Once isolated, the deciduum can be classified into ventral (usually narrower and lighter) and dorsal (larger and darker) ends. The unfixed deciduum is placed into fresh buffer and then pinched in the middle with very fine forceps to separate the ventral end from the dorsal. The E8–E10 embryo in the ventral end can be obtained by gently pulling apart the ventral deciduum. It should still be surrounded by the yolk sac and amnion. These membranes can be removed by tearing them with forceps. The embryo is transferred into fixative (Section 2.3.1.4) using an autoclaved toothpick or a sterile Pasteur pipette.

Older embryos (E11–E20) can be excised directly from the uterus by cutting open the myometrium and popping out an embryo within its yolk sac which can be torn or cut open. After rinsing, the embryo is placed on its side on aluminium foil. Excess buffer is carefully removed with the edge of a tissue or the tip of a triangular piece of filter paper before the embryo is frozen on dry ice.

2.3.1.4 Prefixing and embedding E8–E10 tissue

For early stages, prefixation and sucrose infiltration produce better tissue preservation and facilitate sectioning. Later stages do not need to be prefixed as the tissue integrity is tighter and can be manipulated as in the standard protocol (Chapter 1). E8–E10 decidua or embryos are transferred to an Eppendorf tube of fixative (see Chapter 1) for 5 min and to another for 25 min. The tissues are transferred to PBS for 1 min and then to sucrose (0.5 M in DEPC-treated PBS, pH 7.4) until they sink to the bottom (approx. 30 min). This is followed by a further rinse in PBS. The decidua, after being frozen on dry ice, can be embedded and sectioned. Fixed E8–E10 embryos must be embedded unfrozen. An embedding chamber (e.g. Peel-a-Way disposable embedding moulds no. 18985; Polysciences) is one-third filled with embedding fluid (e.g. Tissue-Tec, O.C.T. Compound no. 4583; Miles). Using a toothpick, several fixed sucrose-infiltrated E8–E10 embryos are placed on the fluid surface. Controlling orientation is difficult as the embryos are very small and tend to break in the viscous fluid. More embedding fluid is gently added on top until the chamber is half-full. After noting the position and depth of the embryos, the chamber is placed into dry ice until the embedding fluid has completely solidified. Such embedded embryos can be stored frozen at −70°C for up to 6 months if wrapped in parafilm. Before sectioning, the plastic chamber is cut away with a razor blade and the tissue block is attached to a cryostat specimen holder. Sections are cut beginning from the top surface.

2.3.2 Postnatal brains

In principle, the techniques required for excision of early postnatal and adult brains are the same. After anaesthetization with CO_2 and decapitation, the head is cooled on ice. The skull sutures at this stage can easily be cut with small scissors. The rear skull plates are removed first, then the brain is cut forwards along the sagittal suture. The young brain is very soft and easily damaged, so the scissor points must be advanced only a few millimetres each snip, and the interior blade must be kept horizontal to the brain surface. Once the frontal skull plate has been cut, the skull plates are folded back with forceps. If the meninges are not torn off with the bone, they must be carefully removed from the brain surface with forceps and fine scissors, otherwise they can cut through the brain on its removal like a cheesewire. The brain is carefully scooped out with a narrow (5 mm) spatula, beginning at the front and working back, allowing the brain to drop gently on to aluminium foil. The brain is frozen on dry ice.

2.4 SECTIONING TIPS

All tissues should be allowed to equilibrate to the cutting temperature (−22 to −24°C) for 1 h before sectioning, otherwise section compression, expansion or fracturing can readily occur. It is useful to stain occasional sections while cutting to identify structures and orientation (Figure 2.1). The air-dried section is dipped in thionin stain (Chapter 1, Protocol 1.9, step 14) for a few seconds, then rinsed in water. After cutting, *all* sections should be fixed and dehydrated as described in Chapter 1, Protocol 1.2.

Three orientations are possible when sectioning the whole uterus, using the mesometrium as a reference point (see Rugh, 1991). When embedding the frozen deciduum, it should be orientated with the ventral pole to the top to obtain transverse sections of the embryo. Sectioning the deciduum vertically gives longitudinal embryo sections. However, excision and freezing may alter the embryo position, so these are only approximate orientations.

Staining of parallel sections to check position and orientation is essential when cutting early embryos (E8–E10), as they are invisible in the white embedding compound (Figure 2.1A). When coronal or sagittal sections of later embryos (E11–E20) are being cut, they should be orientated head downwards (i.e. knife begins cutting section at the head) as this minimizes damage to the brain and surrounding tissues (Figure 2.1B).

2.5 HYBRIDIZATION TROUBLESHOOTING

All slide-mounted embryo sections should be hybridized as described for adult brain sections (Chapter 1, Protocol 1.5 and 1.6) (Figure 2.2). Some additional points are worth noting.

2.5.1 Non-specific hybridization

2.5.1.1 Peripheral tissues

Non-specific hybridization often occurs on peripheral embryonic tissues (Figures 2.3A and 2.3B). Different oligonucleotide probes show different degrees of this, and it is therefore necessary always to perform controls in which excess unlabelled probe is added to the hybridization buffer (see Chapter 1, Protocol 1.5, footnote *a*).

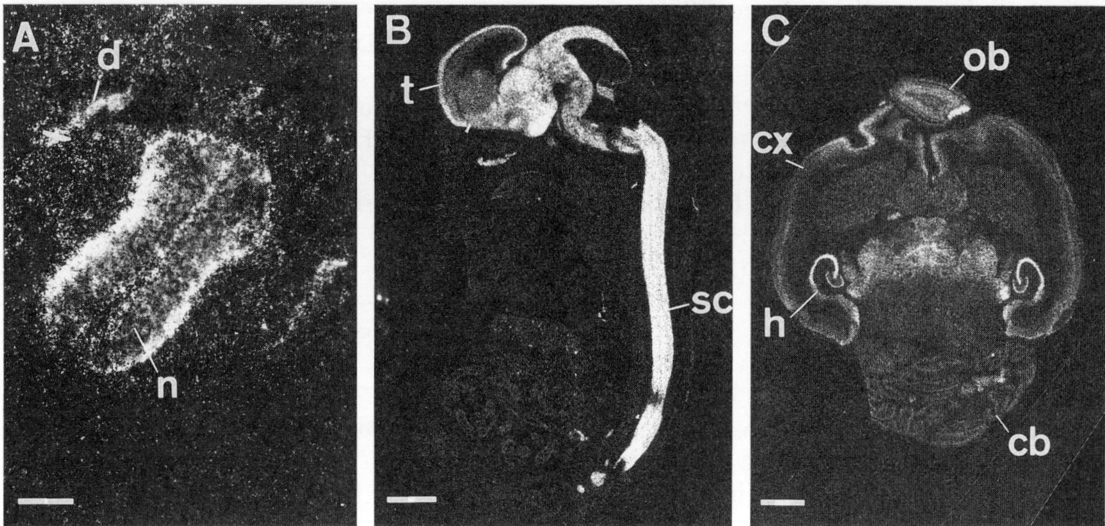

Figure 2.2 *In situ* hybridization signals. (A) Prefixed mouse E9.5 embryo (Nestin probe, darkfield photomicrograph) (data provided by P.C.U. Schrotz and W.B. Huttner), (B) rat E17 embryo (GABA$_A$ receptor β$_3$ subunit probe) and (C) rat P6 brain (GABA$_A$ receptor α$_2$ subunit probe). Abbreviations: d, dorsal root; n, neural tube; others as for Figure 2.1. Bars = 0.1 mm (A) and 2 mm (B and C).

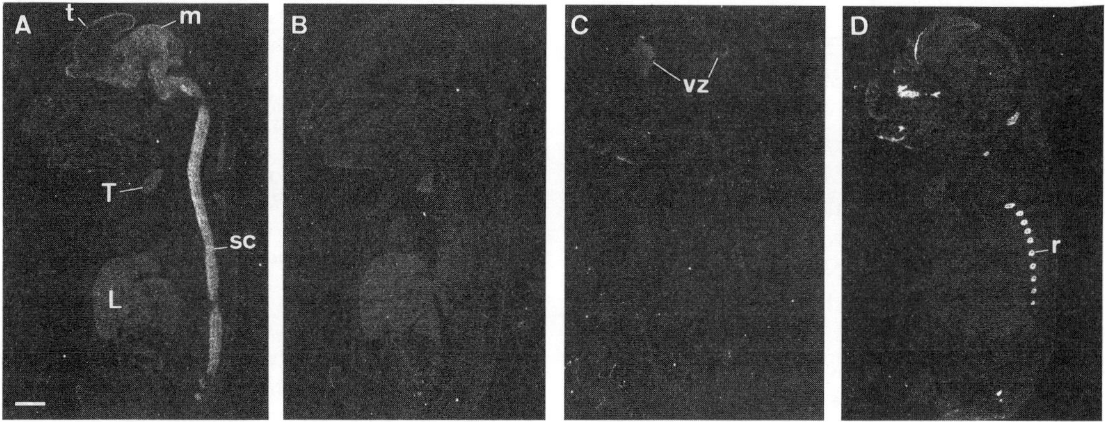

Figure 2.3 Illustration of non-specific hybridization problems on rat E19 embryo sections. (A) and (B) Total and non-specific hybridization (competition) signals using an NMDA NR1 (splice variant del1) subunit probe. (C) Non-specific hybridization of an NMDA receptor NR1 (splice variant del1+2) subunit probe which had a long poly(dA) tail. (D) Non-specific hybridization of an NMDA receptor δ$_1$ subunit probe which had a ^{33}P-labelled poly(dA) tail. Abbreviations: L, liver; m, mesencephalon; sc, spinal cord; t, telencephalon; T, thymus; vz, ventricular zone. Bar = 2 mm.

2.5.1.2 Ventricular zones

Proliferative, cell-dense ventricular zones of the embryonic central nervous system (CNS) exhibit the same problems as adult cerebellar granule cells (see Chapter 1, Figure 1.12) in that they non-specifically trap probes with poly(dA) tails which are too long (Figure 2.3C).

2.5.1.3 Drying out

If the section slightly dries out during hybridization or washing, it can markedly increase background signals. This can be avoided by spreading hybridization buffer evenly on the slide, by ensuring no overhang of the parafilm coverslip and by transferring each slide individually into a rack submerged in SSC before washing.

2.5.1.4 [³³P]dATP

The use of [^{33}P]dATP to tail oligonucleotide probes is not recommended for embryonic sections as it appears to result in non-specific labelling of cartilagenous tissue (Figure 2.3D).

2.5.2 Excessive staining

Hybridized embryo and early postnatal sections can be dipped in photographic emulsion and stained exactly as described in Chapter 1, Protocol 1.9 but brief (30 s) stain immersion times should be used. Embryonic tissue binds the dye faster than adult tissue and the Nissl stain should not impede visualization of the silver grains (Figure 2.2A).

2.6 STRUCTURE IDENTIFICATION

The developing mouse brain has been thoroughly mapped (Theiler, 1989; Rugh, 1991; Schambra *et al.*, 1992; Kaufman, 1992). However, at present no comprehensive anatomical atlas exists for the developing rat CNS. Paxinos *et al.* (1991) is currently the best for the rat and gives sagittal (E14) and coronal (E16, E19, P0) maps, while Swanson (1992) gives a few diagrams of early rat embryo CNS. Structures of the postnatal brain can usually be identified by comparison with an adult brain atlas (Paxinos & Watson, 1986; Swanson, 1992).

ACKNOWLEDGEMENTS

These procedures were established in the laboratories of Professor P.H. Seeburg and Professor W. B. Huttner whom the authors thank for support (SFB 317).

REFERENCES

Dunnett, S. & Björklund, A. (1992) In *Neural transplantation – a practical approach.* S.B. Dunnett & A. Björklund (eds). IRL Press, Oxford, pp. 1–19.

Goedbloed, J.F. & Smits-van Prooije, A.E. (1986) *Acta Anat.* **125**, 76–82.

Hogan, B., Costantini, F. & Lacy, E. (1986) *Manipulating the mouse embryo.* Cold Spring Harbor Laboratory Press, Cold Spring Harbor, NY.

Juurlink, B.H.J. & Federoff, S. (1980) *In Vitro* **15**, 86.

Kaufman, M.H. (1992) *The atlas of mouse development.* Academic Press, London.

Laurie, D.J., Wisden, W. & Seeburg, P.H. (1992) *J. Neurosci.* **12**, 4151–4172.

Paxinos, G. and Watson, C. (1986). *The rat brain in stereotaxic coordinates.* 2nd edn. Academic Press, Sydney.

Paxinos, G., Tork, I., Tecott, L.H. & Valentino, K.L. (1991). *Atlas of developing rat brain.* Academic Press, San Diego.

Rugh, R. (1991). *The mouse. Its reproduction and development.* Oxford University Press, Oxford.

Schambra, U.B., Lauder, J.M. & Silver, J. (1992). *Atlas of the prenatal mouse brain.* Academic Press, San Diego.

Swanson, L.W. (1992). *Brain maps. Structure of the rat brain.* Elsevier, Amsterdam.

Theiler, K. (1989). *The house mouse. Atlas of embryonic development.* 2nd edn. Springer-Verlag, New York.

CHAPTER THREE

Logistics of hybridizing/ processing large tissue specimens

D.J.S. SIRINATHSINGHJI

Merck, Sharp and Dohme Research Laboratories, Neuroscience Research Centre, Terlings Park, Harlow, Essex CM20 2QR

3.1 INTRODUCTION

The *in situ* hybridization (ISH) procedures using radiolabelled (for example with [^{35}S]dATP) synthetic deoxyribonucleotide probes as outlined in Chapter 1 are routinely followed in our laboratories to study gene expression patterns in large brain tissue specimens, for example, whole coronal sections of rhesus or cynomolgus monkey brain or blocks of similar size from human brain. The study of the mRNA expression of a specific neuronal marker in such large sections (rather than in several small blocks) is advantageous, as the mRNA labelling is easily visible in several nuclei on the same section thus facilitating qualitative and quantitative comparisons of the specific mRNA signal from nucleus to nucleus and from animal to animal. An appreciation of this advantage may be realized when it is noted that the ISH procedure can easily be performed on whole coronal sections of the brain from animals with a brain width of 50–55 mm such as

young adult (7–10 years old), rhesus or cynomologus monkeys (Figures 3.1 and 3.2) compared with the brain width of 3–4 mm in young adult (3–4 months) male rats. However, it is important to realize that the quality of the hybridization signal in a specific brain area is only as good as the quality of the brain section. Thus great care should be taken during the preparation of the tissues for subsequent sectioning and during cryostat sectioning itself.

3.2 PREPARATION OF BRAIN SECTIONS

As it is practically impossible to mount and section a whole rhesus or cynomolgus monkey brain in a cryostat, it is desirable to take coronal slices of the brain through regions of experimental interest. This can easily be achieved by placing the brain on a flat sterile surface (e.g. the top surface of a sterile Petri dish, Falcon 1058, 150

IN SITU HYBRIDIZATION PROTOCOLS FOR THE BRAIN
ISBN 0–12–759919–3

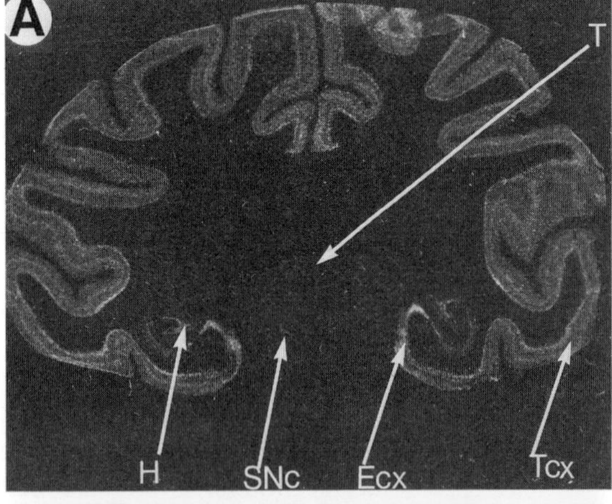

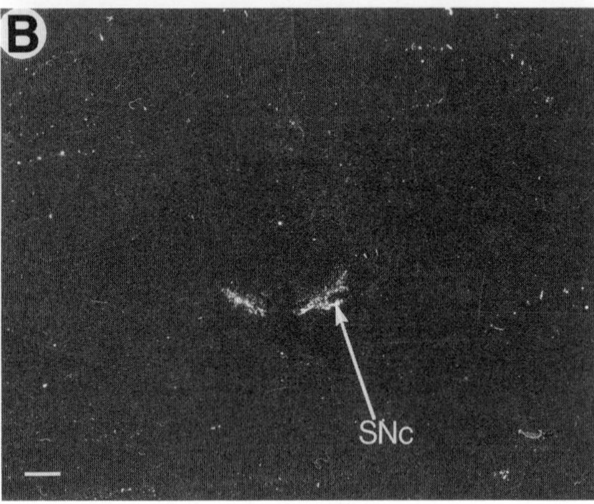

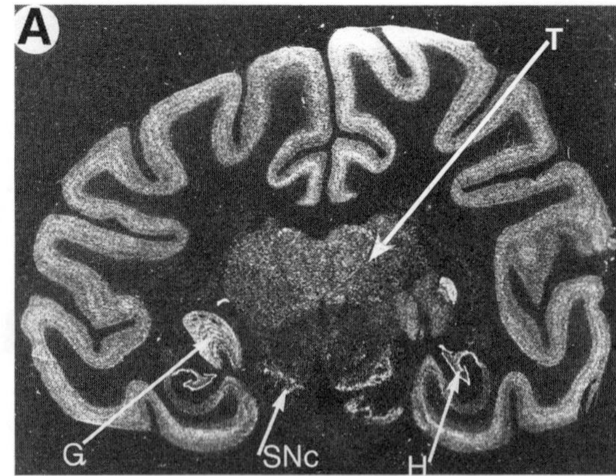

Figure 3.1 The localization of cholecystokinin (CCK) mRNA (A) and tyrosine hydroxylase (TH) mRNA (B) by ISH of adjacent coronal brain sections taken at the level of the ventral mesencephalon of a 17-year-old cynomolgus monkey (*Macaca fascicularis*) with ^{35}S-labelled synthetic 45-mer antisense oligonucleotide probes using the protocols described. The CCK and TH probes were complementary to bases 365–409 of the human CCK gene (Takahashi *et al.*, 1985) and to bases 301–345 of the human TH gene (Grima *et al.*, 1987) respectively. Note the strong and widespread distribution of the CCK mRNA signal in various cortical regions, e.g. the entorhinal (Ecx) and temporal (Tcx) cortices and hippocampus (H) but little or no expression in the thalamic nuclei (T) or pars compacta of the substantia nigra (SNc) and the restricted localization of the TH mRNA labelling in the SNc (B). Exposure time was 5 days on Hyperfilm β_{max}. Scale bar = 500 μm.

Figure 3.2 The localization of the 695-amino acid mRNA transcript of the β-amyloid protein precursor (β-APP$_{695}$) (A) in a whole coronal brain section taken through the hippocampal formation of a 12-year-old rhesus monkey (*Macaca mulatta*) using the described ISH procedures. The section was hybridized with ^{35}S-labelled synthetic 45-mer antisense oligonucleotide probe. The probe was a junctional probe, complementary to bases 966–989 and 1158–1178 (i.e. sequences on either side of the Kunitz protease inhibitor insert) (Ponte *et al.*, 1988). Note the dense hybridization signals in various cortical fields, the thalamus (T), hippocampus (H), lateral geniculate nucleus (G) and pars compacta of the substantia nigra (SNc). Exposure time was 5 days on Hyperfilm β_{max}. The specificity of the antisense probe was verified by the lack of signal on hybridization of an adjacent coronal brain section with ^{35}S-labelled sense β-APP$_{695}$ probe complementary to the sequence of the antisense probe (B). Scale bar = 500 μm.

× 15 mm) and coronal slices (2 cm thick or less) cut with a sharp sterile blade. To obtain a flat even surface at least on one side of the brain slice which is useful for later cryostat sectioning, the brain slice can be placed on the inside surface of a Petri dish and frozen on solid CO_2 (dry ice). When the brain slice is frozen, it should be removed from the dish, wrapped in aluminium foil and stored in a −70°C freezer in air-tight plastic bags. Sections (10–15 μm) are then cut in a cryostat (e.g. Bright Instruments, UK; model OTF/AS-001 or Reichert Frigocut 2800) and mounted on to large glass slides (76 × 50 mm) (Chance) which have been sterilized by baking at 180°C for at least 4 h and coated with poly(L-lysine) (see Protocol 1.1, Chapter 1). Note that one of these slides can accommodate only one coronal section of a rhesus or cynomolgus monkey brain and only two from a squirrel monkey brain. The sections are fixed in 4% paraformaldehyde and stored in 95% ethanol at +4°C as described in Protocol 1.2 (Chapter 1).

However, because of the high lipid content in such large sections which may bind probe non-specifically, we have found it useful to add a delipidation step (with chloroform) during the dehydration step after post-fixation in paraform-aldehyde. Thus, the sequence is as follows: 70% ethanol (5 min), 95% ethanol (5 min), 100% ethanol (5 min), chloroform (5 min), 100% ethanol (5 min) and then storage in 95% ethanol at +4°C.

3.3 LABELLING OF PROBES AND PURIFICATION, HYBRIDIZATION AND POST-HYBRIDIZATION CONDITIONS AND PROCEDURES

The protocols we use for the labelling and purification of labelled probes and the composition of the hybridization buffer are exactly the same as described (Protocols 1.4 and 1.7 respectively, Chapter 1). In addition, as in our experiments, we routinely use probes of lengths varying from 40 to 48 bases, our hybridization and post-hybridization conditions are exactly as described in Chapter 1. However, here are a few modifications which we have found to be necessary for the hybridization of large tissue sections.

(i) Because of the large surface area of the sections, it is advisable to apply about 500 μl of hybridization buffer to each section. We usually apply 300 000–500 000 c.p.m. of the labelled probe/500 μl of hybridization buffer (i.e. 1–2 μl of labelled probe/100 μl of buffer) to each section (see Protocol 1.5, Chapter 1) and cover with parafilm coverslips (70 × 50 mm). Thus, if a large number of such large sections are being run for the same mRNA it may be necessary to perform more than one labelling of the same probe to provide the required probe concentration and radioactivity counts. (ii) We also find that 100 μl of DTT per 1000 μl of hybridization buffer helps to prevent non-specific binding of ^{35}S-labelled probes to large brain sections where lipid content is high.

3.4 X-RAY FILM AND LIQUID EMULSION AUTORADIOGRAPHY

For these procedures, see Sections 1.5 and 1.6 and Protocol 1.9. We routinely use the Amersham Hyperfilm-β_{max} X-ray film (single-sided emulsion) which gives excellent sensitivity and resolution. This film must be developed manually. As regards the liquid emulsion dipping of the large slides (76 × 50 mm), a dipping chamber of equivalent dimensions is obviously necessary. Contact a glass blower!

REFERENCES

Grima, B., Lamouroux, A., Boni, C., Julien, J-F., Javoy-Agid, F. & Mallet, J. (1987) *Nature* **326**, 707–711.

Ponte, P., Gonzalez-DeWhitt, P., Schilling, J., Miller, J., Hsu, D., Greenberg, B., Davis, K., Wallace, W., Lieberburg, I., Fuller, F. & Cordell, B. (1988) *Nature* **331**, 525–527.

Takahashi, Y., Kato, K., Hayashizaki, Y., Wakabayashi, T., Ohtsuka, E., Matsuki, S., Ikehara, M. & Matsubara, K. (1985) *Proc. Natl. Acad. Sci. USA* **82**, 1931–1935.

CHAPTER FOUR

In situ hybridization of astrocytes and neurons cultured *in vitro*

L.A. McNaughton*, C. De Felipe† and S.P. Hunt†

*M.R.C. National Institute for Medical Research, The Ridgeway, Mill Hill, London NW7 1AA. UK
† M.R.C. Laboratory of Molecular Biology, MRC Centre, Hills Rd, Cambridge CB2 2QH, UK

4.1 INTRODUCTION

Owing to the complexity of the nervous system, many advantages are offered by the use of isolated cells in culture. It is possible to obtain pure cell populations and control their growth, differentiation or phenotype depending on the culture conditions (Raff, 1989). Furthermore, cells in culture constitute a powerful tool for the localization and quantification of gene expression in mixed populations of cells. The mechanisms of regulation of gene expression following stimulation can easily be studied in this controlled system (McNaughton & Hunt, 1992). When mixed cultures are required for studies of interactions between different cell types (e.g. astrocytes or Schwann cells with central or peripheral neurons), *in situ* hybridization (ISH) allows the study of the differential gene expression pattern of the two populations in response to a given stimulus (De Felipe *et al.*, 1993).

In this chapter we describe techniques for the localization of mRNAs in primary cultures of neurons and glial cells, using ^{35}S-labelled oligonucleotide probes. We limit our chapter to the special issue of methodology for ISH to astrocytes, Schwann cells or neurons in culture. However, the method can also be applied to other cell types grown in culture. We do not discuss the probe labelling, hybridization buffer or washing conditions as these are referred to in detail in Chapter 1.

We use two methods: (i) the growth of cells on glass coverslips and (ii) the growth of cells in chambers mounted on to glass slides (Lab-Tek/Gibco chamber/slide, supplied by Lab-Tek Division, Miles Laboratories, Inc., 30W475 North Aurora Road, Naperville, IL 60540, USA). There are advantages and disadvantages in the use of the Lab-Tek chamber/slides or the traditional coverslips. The tissue culture chambers are costly in comparison with ordinary coverslips, although they are very much easier to handle, because, after the culturing period, they can be treated and manipulated like slides

IN SITU HYBRIDIZATION PROTOCOLS FOR THE BRAIN
ISBN 0–12–759919–3

with brain sections on them (see Chapter 1). The Lab-Tek chambers also enable one to differentially stimulate different groups of cells on the same slide, add different substances to one chamber of each cell type (see McNaughton & Hunt, 1992), and also enable the simultaneous hybridization of different probes to the same slide. However, in our hands, some neuronal cell types such as dorsal root ganglion cells are difficult to grow in the Lab-Tek chambers. In this case, we recommend the use of traditional glass coverslips.

4.2 HYBRIDIZATION PROCEDURES FOR LAB-TEK TISSUE CULTURE CHAMBER/SLIDES

Astrocytes are isolated as described by Lim *et al.* (1990) and plated on to poly-L-lysine (Sigma; catalogue number P9155) or poly-DL-ornithine (Sigma; catalogue number P8638)-coated *glass* tissue culture chamber/slides (Lab-Tek/Gibco). *Glass* slides must be used, as plastic ones will dissolve in the Histoclear or xylene used for coverslipping them. Further, plastic slides sometimes float out of the carrying racks to the surface of the processing solutions making them very difficult to handle and store. Before the cells are plated, the wells should be coated with 100 μl of poly-DL-ornithine or poly-L-lysine and left for 2 h at room temperature. They are then rinsed twice with 1 × PBS and the cells are plated. (Poly-DL-ornithine at 0.01% is dissolved in 0.15 M sodium borate buffer pH 8.4. This solution can be kept at 4°C for several months. Poly-L-lysine can be made up in water as stock and kept frozen at −20°C for months.)

For our particular experiments (see McNaughton & Hunt, 1992), the cells are usually grown for 8–10 days before they are challenged with the different stimuli. The Lab-Tek culture chamber/slides come with two, four or eight

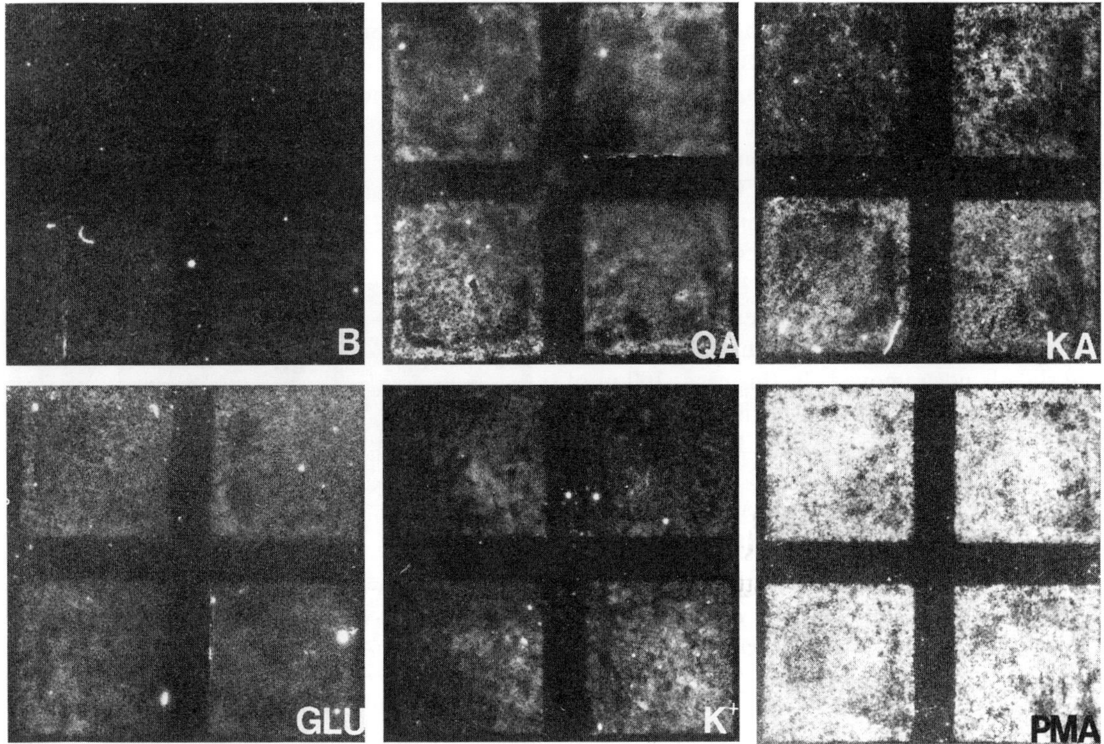

Figure 4.1 A darkfield photomicrograph of cultured astrocytes hybridized with a c-*fos*-specific oligonucleotide. Treatments were as follows; B, unstimulated; QA, quisqualic acid, 100 μM ; KA, kainic acid, 100 μM; Glu, glutamic acid, 100 μM; K⁺, 140 μM; PMA, phorbol ester, 200 nM (see McNaughton & Hunt, 1992). Reproduced with permission from Elsevier Science Publishers.

chambers/wells mounted on to each glass slide. Thus, different treatments or stimuli can be applied to the same slide (Figure 4.1) and consequently processed in parallel, so that intra-assay variations are minimized. For most of our studies, 20–30 min of stimulation with excitatory amino acid was long enough to see changes in immediate early gene expression for cells in culture (see Figure 4.1 and McNaughton & Hunt, 1992). However, 12–24 h or longer stimulations have also been carried out (De Felipe *et al.*, 1993).

After the culture period, the plastic walls and seal that compartmentalize the slide can be easily removed according to the manufacturer's instructions and the slide is ready to be processed in exactly the same way as slides with brain sections using the staining troughs and racks illustrated in Chapter 1 (Figure 1.2); i.e. the slides are rinsed in 250 ml of DEPC-treated 1 × PBS (see Chapter 1, Protocol 1.2, footnote *c*, for PBS recipe). Cells are then fixed for 5 min in 250 ml of cold 4% paraformaldehyde in 1 × PBS. After the fixation the cells are rinsed in 250 ml of PBS followed by dehydration through graded alcohols (Chapter 1, Protocol 1.2). This procedure is carried out at room temperature. Samples are ready to be hybridized or alternatively can be stored long-term in 95% ethanol at 4°C until required for hybridization (see Chapter 1). For the hybridization, 100 µl of hybridization buffer per probe per slide is added with a parafilm coverslip (Chapter 1, Protocol 1.5).

Alternatively, different probes can be used in the same slide if the upper structure which divides the slide is not removed. In this case, 100 µl of the probe hybridization buffer is added to each well. No parafilm is necessary. Hybridization is performed for 20–24 h at 42°C (Chapter 1, Protocol 1.5, for probe concentration and hybridization buffer). After hybridization, the chambers can be removed from the slides and they can be washed as normal (Chapter 1, Protocol 1.6).

4.3 HYBRIDIZATION PROCEDURES FOR GLASS COVERSLIPS

Adult sensory neurons are isolated as described by Lindsay (1988) and plated on to poly-L-lysine or poly-DL-ornithine-coated 19 mm round glass coverslips (BDH/Merck no. 1) which are placed in 12-well plates (made by Linbro or Costar). As for the Lab-Tek slides, *glass* coverslips must be used as plastic ones will dissolve in the Histoclear or xylene used for coverslipping them. Laminin, (Sigma; catalogue number L-2020), an alternative substrate used in some neuronal cultures, does not interfere with the ISH technique and therefore can be used if needed.

Throughout the procedure, coverslips are manipulated by the combined action of a pair of fine forceps and a fine needle (e.g. syringe or mounting pin), the needle being used to help tease and lift the coverslips from the bottom of the well. They are generally not removed from the wells, and solutions (usually between 3 and 4 ml per well) are pipetted on to and aspirated off them. In the cases where the coverslips are removed, for example in order to dry them after ethanol storage or after the post-hybridization washing steps, they can be placed in the type of rack illustrated in Figure 4.2.

Before plating and culturing of the cells, the coverslips are washed in HCl (0.5 M) for 1 h, after which they are rinsed in copious distilled water with a final rinse in absolute (100%) ethanol. The coverslips are allowed to dry, wrapped in aluminium foil and sterilized by

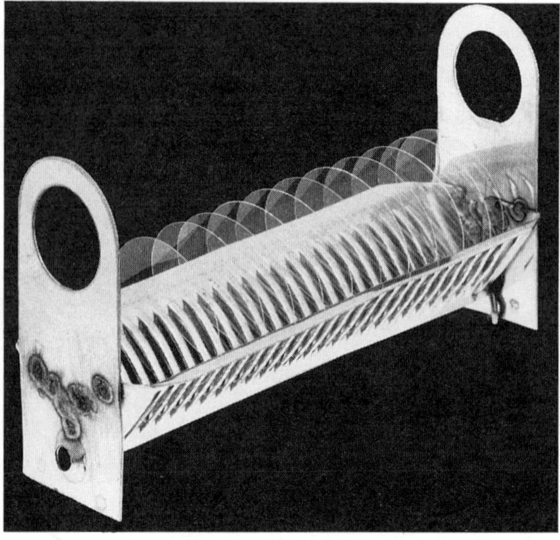

Figure 4.2 Illustration of the type of rack used for holding the glass cell culture coverslips.

baking for 2 h at 180°C. The washed coverslips are placed in 12-well plates using forceps. Then 1 ml per well of 0.01% poly-DL-ornithine is added, and the coverslips are left for 2 h at room temperature followed by a rinse with 1 × PBS. Then 0.5 ml of laminin (5 µg ml^{-1} in 1 × PBS stocked in aliquots at −70°C) is immediately added, and the mixture incubated at 37°C for 3 or 4 h. The laminin is aspirated (the coverslips must not be rinsed) and the cells are plated on.

After the culture period, the coverslips are rinsed in 2 ml of DEPC-treated 1 × PBS. Cells are then fixed for 5 min in 2 ml of cold 4% paraformaldehyde in 1 × PBS (Chapter 1). After fixation, the cells are rinsed in 1 × PBS followed by dehydration through graded alcohol. At each stage, 2 ml of each solution is pipetted on to and then aspirated from the coverslips. At no point are the coverslips removed from the wells. This procedure is carried out at room temperature. Samples are ready to be hybridized or stored in 95% or absolute ethanol at 4°C (Chapter 1, Protocol 1.2). For long-term storage, 3 or 4 ml of ethanol is pipetted into each well. The lid is sealed with parafilm, and the plates placed at 4°C.

Before hybridization, coverslips are removed from the dish and air-dried in a rack (Figure 4.2) in a dust-free environment at room temperature for 30 min. The coverslips are then placed back in a new clean sterilized 12-well plate where the next steps of hybridization and washing are actually carried out.

The probe to be hybridized is added in 50 µl of hybridization buffer (probe concentration and hybridization buffer composition as in Chapter 1) and pipetted on to the coverslips. This is then covered with hand-cut parafilm coverslips cut into small circles, avoiding the formation of air bubbles between the coverslip and the slide. The dishes are incubated at 42°C in a humidified atmosphere for 18–20 h. It is important to leave at least two empty wells in the dish and to add distilled water to them. This keeps a humidified atmosphere in the dish. Any dehydration of the sample will cause erratic and false results because the hybridization and washes are carried out in an air incubator.

After hybridization, covering the coverslips with liquid makes them much easier to remove, therefore 4 ml of prewarmed 1 × SSC (55°C) is pipetted into each well before removal of the parafilm coverslips. Then, by combined teasing with forceps and a syringe needle, the parafilm coverslips can be easily removed. The wells are placed in an air incubator set at the washing temperature (55°C). After half an hour, the SSC is changed by aspiration, and another 4 ml of preheated 1 × SSC is pipetted into each well. After the final washing step, the coverslips are removed one at a time from the wells with forceps and needle and dipped sequentially into 0.1 × SSC, 70% ethanol and 95% ethanol. The coverslips are air-dried in racks (Figure 4.2).

With the cells facing up, the coverslips are then attached to a cleaned histology slide by using DPX (BDH) as glue, so that the slides can be either exposed to X-ray film (Kodak, Figure 4.3)

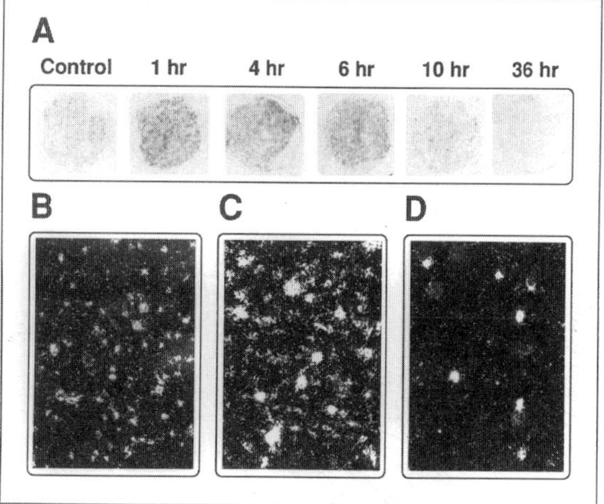

Figure 4.3 Dissociated adult rat dorsal root ganglion cells growing on 19 mm coverslips. Cells were treated with cycloheximide, fixed at different times and hybridized with ^{35}S-labelled c-*jun* antisense oligonucleotide. (A) Autoradiograph image of the coverslips. (B), (C) and (D) silver grains over neurons (large cells) and Schwann cells (small cells) under darkfield illumination in control cells (B) or after 2 h (C) or 12 h (D) of treatment respectively. c-*jun* mRNA was increased from 1 to 8 h of treatment in both cell types. After 10 h of treatment and onwards c-*jun* expression disappeared in Schwann cells but not in neurons (see De Felipe *et al.*, in preparation).

and/or dipped in emulsion (Figures 4.1 and 4.3). X-ray film is very useful for macroscopic observations and quantification of hybridization with radiolabelled oligonucleotide probes, where different levels of expression can be assessed by densitometry (see Chapter 7). When a more detailed and fine analysis is needed, dipping for autoradiography in photographic emulsions is the method of choice (Chapter 1, Protocol 1.9 and Chapter 5, Section 5.4.2). The final thionin staining allows identification of the cellular localization of the silver grains.

REFERENCES

De Felipe, C., Jenkins, R., O'Shea R., Williams, T.S.C. & Hunt, S.P. (1993) *Adv. Neurol.* **59**, 263–271.

Lim, R. & Bosch, E.P. (1990) In *Methods in Neurosciences*, Vol. 2, *Cell culture*, P.M. Conn (ed.). Academic Press, New York.

Lindsay, R.M. (1988) *J. Neurosci.* **8**, 2394–2405.

McNaughton, L.A. & Hunt, S.P. (1992) *Mol. Brain. Res.* **16**, 261–266.

Raff, M.C. (1989) *Science* **243**, 1450–1455.

CHAPTER FIVE

In situ hybridization on organotypic slice cultures

A. GERFIN-MOSER* & H. MONYER†

* Brain Research Institute, August-Forel Str. 1, CH-8029 Zurich, Switzerland † Centre for Molecular Boiology (ZMBH), Im Neuenheimer Feld 282, D-69120 Heidelberg, Germany

5.1 INTRODUCTION

Slice cultures of nervous tissue represent an *in vitro* preparation that is thin enough to use for experimental manipulations and visualization of individual cells, yet retains much of the basic structural and connective organization of its tissue of origin (Gähwiler, 1981). In culture, the slices become thinned to a quasi-monolayer, facilitating study of the single cells that form the intricate neuronal network. Organotypic neuronal cultures can be derived from various brain regions. The cytoarchitectural organization of the parent slice is retained and the spatial distribution of synaptic connections, which develop '*de novo*' during the first weeks in culture, forms much as it would *in situ*. As an *in vitro* analogue of axonal connectivities between brain areas, slices from regions that are anatomically remote but interconnected in the brain can be cocultured, providing a powerful model for studying the development and function of neuronal projections

(Gähwiler *et al.*, 1991). Organotypic cultures thus offer several advantages over other preparations, such as cultures of dissociated cells or acute slices, and are well suited for acute and long-term pharmacological, electrophysiological and morphological studies. For example, it is of interest to study changes in gene expression associated with chronic epilepsy (Müller *et al.*, 1993; Moser *et al.*, 1993), growth factors (Gähwiler *et al.*, 1987) or developmental changes in the culture system (Finsen *et al.*, 1992).

In situ hybridization (ISH) allows the visualization of gene expression in cells at the mRNA level. Each cell represents a living single unit within a highly organized network, which can be investigated under standard culture conditions and also after a variety of experimental manipulations. In this chapter we illustrate the use of the ISH technique, based on the procedure described in Chapter 1 and adapted for organotypic neuronal cultures. We have used probes for several ligand-gated ion-channel receptor subunits on rat hippocampal slice cultures which were

IN SITU HYBRIDIZATION PROTOCOLS FOR THE BRAIN
ISBN 0–12–759919–3

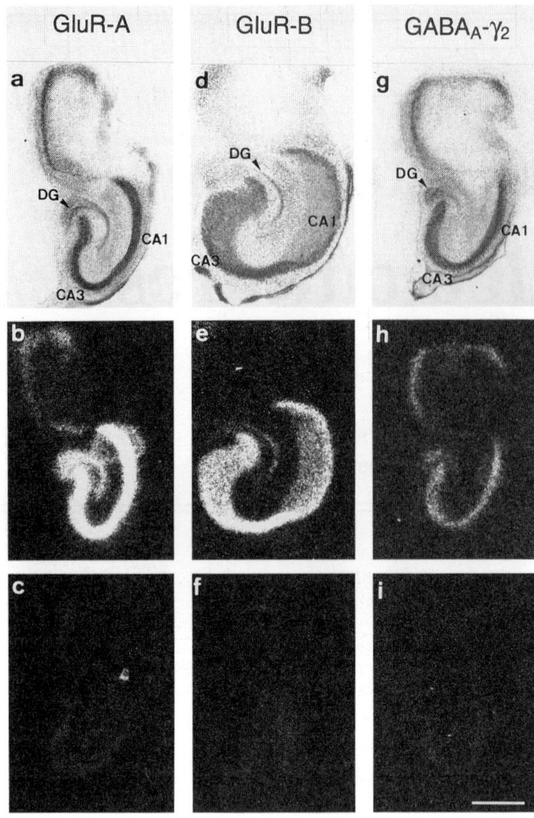

Figure 5.1 Detection of mRNAs encoding subunits A and B of the AMPA-selective glutamate receptor and subunit γ_2 of the GABA$_A$ receptor in hippocampal slice culture preparations. Nissl stains of cultures hybridized with the labelled probe (a, d and g) demonstrate the morphological variability of the cultured hippocampi. The corresponding X-ray films (b, e, h) show the mRNA levels for each receptor subunit present in these cultures. The signals are displaced by adding excess unlabelled oligonucleotides to the probe as visualized by the X-ray films in c, f and i. Exposure time was 5 days for GluR-A and -B and 7 days for GABA$_A$-γ_2. The same magnification was used for all images, Bar in i = 1 mm. DG, dentate gyrus.

allowed to mature under standard conditions for 2–3 weeks. The cultures were kindly provided by the laboratory of Dr B. H. Gähwiler at the Brain Research Institute in Zurich. We chose oligonucleotide probes not only because they allow for subunit specificity but also because they yield lower non-specific labelling than cRNA probes. This latter point was particularly important with respect to the labelling obtained in the pyramidal cell regions of the hippocampal cultures as they

maintained a thickness of 2–3 cell layers. The hybridization pattern was revealed by exposure to X-ray film or autoradiographic emulsion as stated.

As shown in Figure 5.1 (a, d, g), Nissl staining revealed a certain variability in the shape of the cultured hippocampal formation due to various amounts of cell migration and flattening of the culture compared with the size and shape of the original slice. Hybridization with probes for the AMPA-selective glutamate receptor subunits A or B of the rat (GluR-A, GluR-B) (Keinänen *et al.*, 1990; Boulter *et al.*, 1990) gave a strong signal in all hippocampal areas for both probes, as shown by the corresponding images of the X-ray film (Figure 5.1b, e). On the other hand, labelling of the cells with a probe specific for the subunit γ_2 of the GABA$_A$ receptor resulted in a much fainter image of the hippocampal formation, although the specific radioactivity of the probe used was similar to those for GluR-A and -B and the exposure to X-ray film was 2 days longer (7 days; Figure 5.1h). In this case, the relative signal intensities corresponded roughly to what would be expected from comparison with data obtained in brain sections (Werner *et al.*, 1991; Killisch *et al.*, 1991). Control hybridization of cultures with a mixture containing the radioactively labelled probe and an excess of the unlabelled oligonucleotide suppressed signals almost completely for all three probes (Figures 5.1c, f, i), thus highlighting the specificity of binding for the labelled probes.

An example of the regionally selective gene expression in the culture system, which is very similar to observations *in vivo*, is shown in Figure 5.2. Hybridization with a probe for subunit 1 of the kainate-sensitive glutamate receptor (KA-1) yielded an expression pattern that was mainly restricted to the CA3 region of the hippocampus (Figure 5.2b). In contrast, labelling of both CA3 and CA1 (Figure 5.2f) was obtained with a probe for subunit 2 (KA-2) of this receptor (Herb *et al.*, 1992). The weak labelling in the dentate gyrus, compared with *in vivo* expression patterns, probably results from the radiation-induced loss of granule cells (see Section 5.2). Brightfield images of the Nissl stain in Figures 5.2c and 5.2g correspond to X-ray images of control cultures hybridized with excess unlabelled oligonucleotides (Figures 5.2d and 5.2h).

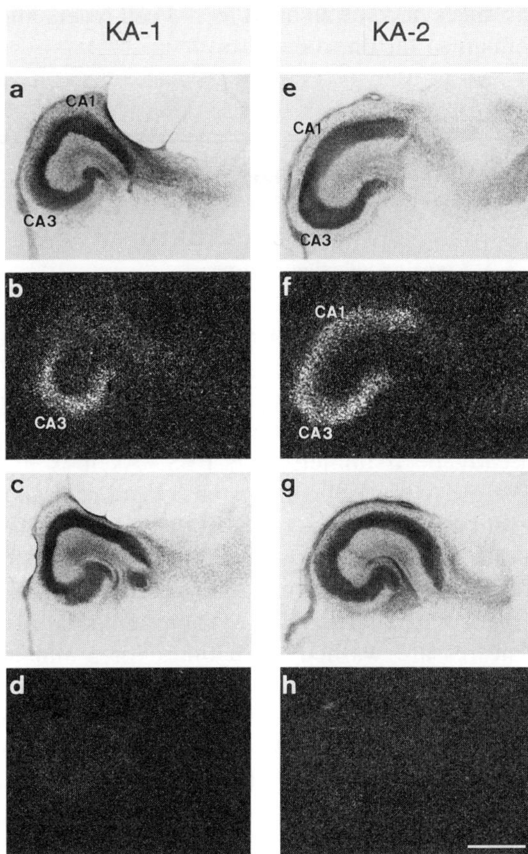

Figure 5.2 *In situ* hybridization of hippocampal slice cultures to demonstrate the regionally selective expression of mRNA encoding the KA-1 subunit of the kainate-sensitive glutamate receptor. The signal on X-ray film obtained with the probe for KA-1 is restricted to the hippocampal CA3 region (b), whereas for KA-2, another subunit of this receptor family, mRNA levels are high in both the CA1 and the CA3 regions (f). Brightfield images show the Nissl stains corresponding to the cultures hybridized with probe (a, e) and to those hybridized with a mixture of probe and excess unlabelled oligonucleotides (c, g). The signal was displaced by addition of unlabelled probes as shown in the X-ray images of these control cultures (d, h). Bar in h = 1 mm.

In order to obtain images of the hybridization pattern at higher cellular resolution, hybridized slice cultures were coated with autoradiographic emulsion. Excellent cellular resolution can be obtained in regions where slices have flattened down to a single cell layer. For example, cerebellar slice cultures are especially well suited for emulsion autoradiography because tissue of cortical origin is almost always thinned to a

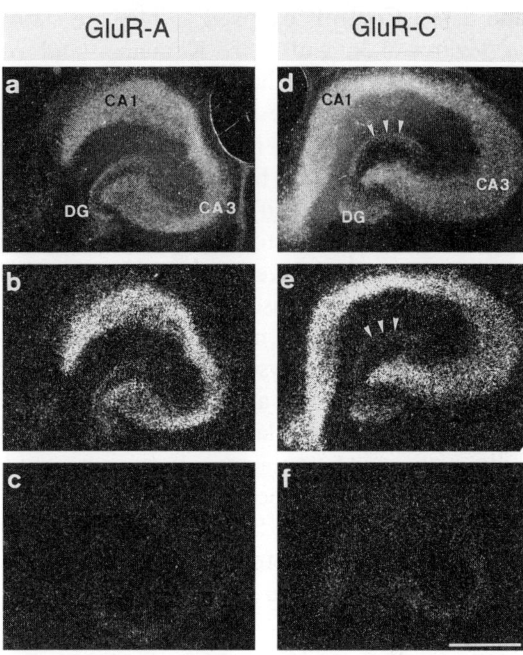

Figure 5.3 Expression of mRNA in hippocampal slice cultures encoding the GluR-A and -C subunit of the AMPA-selective glutamate receptor as revealed by autoradiography on photographic emulsion and X-ray film. For both probes, exposure of the hybridized cultures to emulsion resulted in images of higher resolution and sensitivity (a and d) than in those obtained from exposing the same cultures to X-ray film (b and e). Control cultures were incubated with a mixture of labelled and excess unlabelled oligonucleotides to demonstrate specificity by displacement of the X-ray signal (c and f). Exposure time was 9 days for emulsion and 4 days for X-ray film. Arrowheads indicate the signal in the dentate gyrus (DG) which was weaker when the culture was exposed to X-ray film than when it was exposed to emulsion. Bar in f = 1 mm.

monolayer (data not shown). The difference in resolution between exposure to film or emulsion can be appreciated in Figure 5.3. mRNA expression in hippocampal cultures for GluR-A and GluR-C, two subunits of the AMPA-selective glutamate receptor family (Keinänen *et al.*, 1990; Boulter *et al.*, 1990), was investigated. Hybridized cultures were first exposed to X-ray film for 4 days and then to emulsion for 9 days with the results shown in Figures 5.3a and 5.3d. The higher resolution obtained with emulsion is most conspicuous in the dentate gyrus. A portion of the signal in this area is much weaker or even missing (arrowheads) on X-ray film (Figures 5.3b and 5.3e). Controls exposed to film are shown in Figures 5.3c and 5.3f. Keinänen and co-workers (1990) have shown that mRNA levels for GluR-C within the hippocampal formation in sections from adult rat brain are highest in CA1 and dentate gyrus but diminish significantly in CA3. It can be seen from Figures 5.3a and 5.3b that it is difficult to draw conclusions with regard to the relative amounts of mRNA between regions because the regional thickness of the cultures may not be the same. For semiquantitative analysis silver grains would have to be counted and normalized to the thickness of the cell layer or the number of cells.

The following protocol for ISH focuses on steps that have been adapted for investigations on organotypic slice cultures and thus differ from the detailed description in Chapter 1.

5.2 PREPARATION OF SLICE CULTURES

Slice cultures of rat hippocampus are prepared and maintained *in vitro* as described in detail elsewhere (Gähwiler, 1984; Gähwiler *et al.*, 1991). Briefly, 5–7-day-old rat pups are killed by decapitation. The hippocampus is isolated, 425-µm-thick sections are cut on a tissue chopper under sterile conditions and exposed to ionizing radiation (650 rad, 4.5 min) in order to reduce the number of non-neuronal cells. It should be noted that, because some dentate gyrus cells are still dividing at the time of explantation, irradiation considerably reduces the size of the dentate gyrus in the cultures. The sections are mounted on glass coverslips (12 × 24 mm) in a droplet of clotted chicken plasma (Cocalico), placed in sealed culture tubes containing 0.75 ml of semisynthetic culture medium, and incubated on a slowly rotating roller drum at 36°C. This rotation serves the purpose of providing proper draining, feeding and aeration of the cultures, but also facilitates the gradual flattening and spreading of the slices. The medium consists of 25% horse serum, 50% Eagle's basal medium and 25% of either Hanks' or Earle's balanced salt solution (Gibco). After 17–20 days *in vitro*

the slices become thinned to 1–3 cell layers and remain so far up to 6 weeks.

5.3 *IN SITU* HYBRIDIZATION

5.3.1 Fixation of slice cultures

Briefly, cultures are taken out of the culturing tube with curved fine pointed tweezers and placed in a Teflon rack (custom made) holding 20 coverslips in vertical position which has already been immersed in PBS. As it is not possible to mark the unfrosted coverslips, notes must be taken on the order of the cultures. The rack is transferred into 4% formaldehyde in PBS, freshly prepared from paraformaldehyde, and left for 5 min for fixation at room temperature. Cultures are washed three times for 5 min in PBS, dehydrated in 75% and 95% ethanol for 5 min each and air-dried at room temperature for about 45 min. Racks with cultures that are not to be used immediately for hybridization are placed in a staining trough or wrapped in aluminium foil and stored at −20°C until required. They can be stored in the freezer for up to a couple of weeks without any notable loss of quality in subsequent ISH experiments.

Long-term storage in 95% ethanol at 4°C should be avoided because the alcohol will cause the cultures to come off the coverslip during the washing procedure after the hybridization step, presumably as a result of some effect on the plasma clot that is used in the preparation of the slice cultures.

5.3.2 Hybridization

Frozen cultures are allowed to come to room temperature for 30 min. ^{35}S-labelled probes are diluted in 'minimalist' hybridization buffer as described in Chapter 1. However, probes exceeding 300 000 c.p.m. μl^{-1} are still used for the following reason: as determined by polyacrylamide gel electrophoresis (data not shown), a higher number of counts, obtained by liquid-scintillation counting, does not result from longer AMP tails (more than 50 nucleotides), but rather from a higher number of oligonucleotides carrying a radioactive tail. Probes above 300 000 d.p.m. μl^{-1} are therefore diluted to around 200 000 d.p.m. μl^{-1} with 1× TE buffer. They are not found to produce non-specific binding.

Coverslips are placed horizontally and 30 µl of the hybridization mixture is placed on to each culture. This is sufficient to cover the whole hippocampal region and spreading of the mix is therefore not necessary. A glass slide (baked at 180°C for 3 h) is then gently lowered over the culture until the coverslip attaches to it by adhesion. The slide is inverted and placed horizontally with the culture now sitting on top of it. This way, up to four cultures with application of the same probe can be attached to one slide and its frosted end can be marked with pencil. There is usually no problem of air bubbles. To perform the hybridization, large slide-storage boxes (Kartell, Milano, Italy; 100 slides/box) containing tissues soaked with 10 ml of solution (4×SSC/50% formamide) are used as humidifying chambers. Up to 14 slides (i.e. up to 56 cultures) can be placed horizontally per box. The boxes are sealed with electrical tape to maintain humidity and incubated at 42°C overnight in an oven.

5.3.2.2 *Washing*

Slides are removed from the humidifying chamber and lowered at an angle into a jar containing 2×SSC at 50°C with the coverslips facing downwards. In this way, the coverslips slide off the slides easily and are prevented from landing culture side down on the bottom of the staining jar. The jar should be placed on a black surface to outline the delicate coverslips for easier handling. The cultures are transferred one-by-one back into a Teflon rack immersed in 1×SSC at room temperature. The order of the hybridized cultures must be noted separately. The rack is transferred into prewarmed 1×SSC at 60°C and left for 20 min. A series of rinses at room temperature is then performed for 5 min each: 1×SSC, 0.1×SSC, 75% ethanol and 95% ethanol. Cultures are subsequently allowed to air-dry.

5.4 AUTORADIOGRAPHY

5.4.1 Exposure to X-ray film

Dry coverslips are attached to cardboard with scotch tape and exposed to Kodak XAR-5 autoradiographic film for 3 days to 2 weeks depending on the probes used and the efficiency of their tailing. Autoradiographic ^{14}C-labelled micro-scale strips (Amersham) are found to be very convenient for comparison of films exposed for different lengths of time. After exposure, cultures are removed for subsequent counterstaining or exposure to emulsion by gently peeling the tape off.

5.4.2 Exposure to autoradiographic emulsion

5.4.2.1 *Coating with emulsion*

Emulsion (NTB-2, Kodak) is melted in a waterbath at 42°C, and an aliquot is poured into a black film roll container. A glass slide is dipped and checked for air bubbles. When bubbles are present, the emulsion is not touched for another 15 min. Cultures are dipped individually into the undiluted emulsion for about 5 s. White plastic forceps (metal must not be used!) were used for more convenient handling under safelight illumination. Excess emulsion is allowed to drain by gently touching a tissue with the lower end of the coverslip; the coverslips are then placed 'on end' in a plastic rack to dry. They are left in complete darkness for 4 h overnight. Coated coverslips are transferred to Teflon racks with plastic forceps, then racks are placed into light-tight boxes containing a bag of silica gel and stored for exposure at 4°C for the required time (between 5 days and 4 weeks). See Protocol 1.9 for the use of Ilford K5 emulsion.

5.4.2.2 *Developing and counterstaining*

Exposed boxes are allowed to come to room temperature for 1 h. Emulsion-coated coverslips are developed according to the manufacturer's instructions at 15°C. Briefly, cultures are placed in Dektol developer (Kodak; diluted 1:1 in water) for 2 min, rinsed in water for 30 s, fixed in a freshly prepared solution of 30% sodium thiosulphate for 10 min, and rinsed in running tap water for 20 min. For counterstaining, the rack is transferred to a solution of 0.2% Toluidine Blue and left for several minutes. Cultures are then rinsed for 1 min in water, destained in 0.01 M HCl until the emulsion layer is free of blue stain, rinsed in water for 1 min, destained in 70% ethanol until excess staining of the tissue has been removed (10–30 min, depending on the thickness of the cultures and on the time of staining). Cultures are dehydrated in 95% ethanol, twice in 100% ethanol and cleared twice in 100% xylene for 5 min each. Finally, coverslips are mounted culture side down on microscope slides by slowly lowering them on to a drop of mounting medium (Eukitt, Kindler Germany).

ACKNOWLEDGEMENTS

We would like to thank Drs. Scott Thompson and Peter Streit for critical comments on the manuscript. Special thanks are due to Dr. Beat H. Gähwiler for providing the cultures and to Franziska Grogg and Lotty Rietschin for their excellent technical assistance in preparing them. This work was supported by the Swiss National Science Foundation (Grant nos. 31-28652.90 to P. Streit and 31-27641.89 to B.H. Gähwiler) and the Sandoz Research Institute in Berne, Switzerland.

REFERENCES

Boulter, J., Hollmann, M., O'Shea-Greenfield, A., Hartley, M., Deneris, E., Maron, C. & Heinemann, S. (1990) *Science* **249**, 1033–1037.

Finsen, B.R., Tonder, N., Augood, S. & Zimmer, J. (1992) *Neuroscience* **47**, 105–113.

Gähwiler, B.H. (1981) *Neurosci. Methods* **4**, 329–342.

Gähwiler, B.H. (1984) *Neuroscience* **11**, 751–760.

Gähwiler, B.H., Enz, A. & Hefti, F. (1987) *Neurosci. Lett.* **75**, 6–10.

Gähwiler, B.H., Thompson, S.M., Audinat, E. & Robertson, R.T. (1991) In *Culturing nerve cells.* Banker, G. and Goslin, K. (eds). MIT Press, Cambridge, MA. pp. 379–411.

Herb, A., Burnashev, N., Werner, P., Sakmann, B., Wisden, W. & Seeburg, P.H. (1992). *Neuron* **8**, 775–785.

Keinänen, K., Wisden, W., Sommer, B., Werner, P., Herb, A., Verdoorn, T.A., Sakmann, B. & Seeburg, P.H. (1990). *Science* **249**, 556–560.

Killisch, I., Dotti, C.G., Laurie, D.J., Lüddens, H. & Seeburg, P.H. (1991). *Neuron* **7**, 927–936.

Moser, A.M., Müller, M., Gähwiler, B.H., Thompson, S.M. & Streit, P. (1993). *Experientia* **49**, A74.

Müller, M., Gähwiler, B.H., Rietschin, L. & Thompson, S.M. (1993). *Proc. Natl. Acad. Sci. USA* **90**, 257–261.

Werner, P., Voigt, M., Keinänen, K., Wisden, W. & Seeburg, P.H. (1991). *Nature* **351**, 742–744.

CHAPTER SIX

In situ hybridization on *Drosophila* neural tissue using ^{35}S-labelled oligonucleotides

A. ULTSCH

BASF AG, Department of Biotechnology, D 67056 Ludswighafen, Germany

A number of methods for the detection of *Drosophila* mRNA employ tritiated, ^{32}P- or ^{35}S-labelled DNA or RNA probes and require time-consuming pretreatments and prehybridization of tissue sections in order to render gene transcripts accessible to nucleic acid probes (see, for example, Hafen & Levine, 1986). I have found that the *in situ* hybridization (ISH) protocol of Wisden and Morris (Chapter 1) greatly simplifies the study of spatial mRNA distribution in *Drosophila* with regard to probe labelling and treatment of sections. Importantly, this protocol appears to be comparable in both specificity and sensitivity to other ISH techniques for *Drosophila*.

The protocols in Chapter 1 can be followed almost without change when performing ISH on *Drosophila* cryosections. Minor changes include tissue treatment before embedding in cryoglue and sectioning. *Drosophila* larvae should be rinsed in PBS (80 mM Na_2HPO_4, 20 mM NaH_2PO_4, 130 mM NaCl, pH 7.2) and then fixed in PBS containing 4% (w/v) paraformaldehyde.

In contrast, *Drosophila* embryos should be pretreated as detailed in Chapter 10 (Protocol 10.1, steps 1–8). After embedding and freezing, 7 μm sections are cut on a cryostat. No pretreatments other than those detailed in Chapter 1 (Protocol 1.2) are required for *Drosophila* tissue sections.

Figure 6.1 shows a photomicrograph of a sectioned *Drosophila* embryo after ISH of an ^{35}S-labelled antisense oligonucleotide (45-mer) to mRNA and emulsion autoradiography. The oligonucleotide was designed to exon 5 of the homoeotic gene *Antennapedia* (Levine *et al.*, 1983). Heavy labelling marks neural tissue and the observed spatial distribution is identical with that reported previously (Schneuwly *et al.*, 1986).

REFERENCES

Hafen, E. & Levine, M. (1986). In *Drosophila: a practical approach*. D.B. Roberts (ed.). IRL

IN SITU HYBRIDIZATION PROTOCOLS FOR THE BRAIN
ISBN 0–12–759919–3

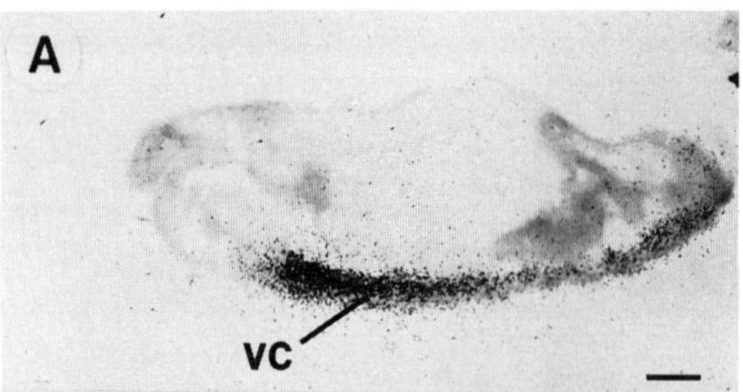

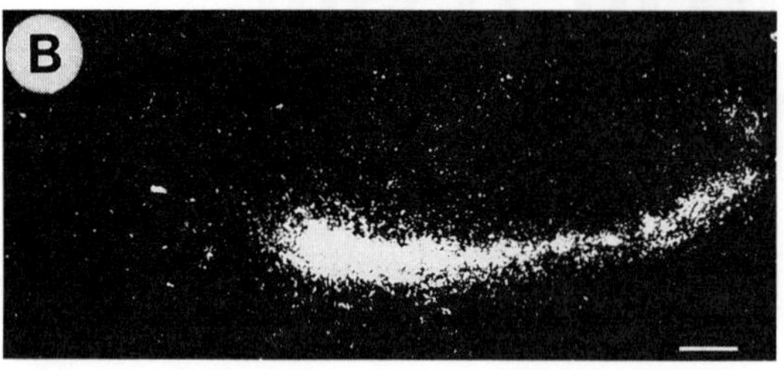

Figure 6.1 *In situ* hybridization of *Antennapedia* transcripts to a ^{35}S-labelled oligonucleotide in a parasagittal tissue cryosection of a late *Drosophila* embryo. Emulsion autoradiography was for 6 weeks. The brightfield (A) and corresponding darkfield (B) photomicrographs show the expression pattern of *Antennapedia* gene transcripts along the developing ventral cord (vc). Scale bar = 50 μm.

Press/Oxford University Press, Oxford. pp. 139–157.

Levine, M., Hafen, E., Garber, R.L. & Gehring, W.J. (1983) *EMBO J.* **2**, 2037–2046.

Schneuwly, S., Kuroiwa, A., Baumgartner, P. & Gehring, W.J. (1986) *EMBO J.* **5**, 733–739.

CHAPTER SEVEN

Quantitative analysis of *in situ* hybridization histochemistry

ROSS D. O'SHEA & ANDREW L. GUNDLACH

University of Melbourne Clinical Pharmacology and Therapeutics Unit, Department of Medicine, Austin and Heidelberg Repatriation Hospitals, Heidelberg, Victoria 3084, Australia

7.1 INTRODUCTION

'A cat may be killed by choking it with cream, but only a few enthusiasts would insist that this is the only available method.' (Rogers, 1979)

Recent advances in several disciplines, including biochemistry, endocrinology and molecular biology, have focused the attention of biological scientists, neuroscientists in particular, on genes that code for specific neuropeptides, enzymes, receptors, and regulatory and structural proteins. This has created a need to understand the control of gene expression. Gene regulation may be studied using a number of molecular biological techniques. Only *in situ* hybridization histochemistry (ISH), however, permits the precise localization of gene expression in a particular tissue, especially in morphologically and functionally complex tissues such as the nervous system (Young, 1990). As changes in gene transcription, indicated by altered levels of mRNA coding for specific peptides or proteins, are physiologically relevant markers of cellular activity (Uhl, 1989; Uhl & Nishimori, 1990), the ability to perceive these changes and to accurately determine their magnitude is of great importance. When comparing levels of mRNA in different anatomical locations, different developmental stages or in response to pharmacological, physiological or surgical manipulations, quantitative analysis of ISH allows not only the identification of localized changes, but measurement of the magnitude of these changes.

Many of the techniques used in the quantitative analysis of ISH are derived from those devised for neurotransmitter receptor autoradiography, the theoretical aspects of which have been reviewed elsewhere (e.g. Kuhar *et al.*, 1986; Davenport & Hall, 1988; Davenport & Nunez, 1990). An understanding of how X-ray films and nuclear emulsions respond to radioactivity is also useful in the design and analysis of ISH experiments; these subjects are excellently

IN SITU HYBRIDIZATION PROTOCOLS FOR THE BRAIN
ISBN 0–12–759919–3

covered in the readable and informative text by Rogers (1979).

The aims of the present chapter are to draw the attention of the reader to the theoretical considerations which should be observed to allow the accurate and meaningful quantification of ISH, and to provide practical advice and instructions for this analysis. We have focused on convenient computerized methods for the quantitative analysis of ISH results, as these are now far more widely used and efficient than older manual methods. The methods of analysis described in this chapter are most relevant to the results of ISH experiments obtained using radioisotopically labelled DNA oligonucleotides which hybridize to mRNA in thin tissue sections, although many of the theoretical aspects of this analysis are of relevance for a wider range of experimental situations.

7.2 GENERAL CONSIDERATIONS

7.2.1 Experimental design

In designing ISH experiments with a view to quantifying results, it is intuitive that the researcher should attempt to eradicate or at least minimize any potential sources of variation between the treatment of different experimental sections. Although identical processing of sections may not be possible in all instances, samples to be analysed concurrently (i.e. those to be directly compared with each other) should ideally be prepared at the same time and processed together, as between-experiment variation contributes most significantly to the overall variability of results (McCabe et al., 1993). For accurate quantification, sources of variation at each step in the preparation and hybridization of sections and in the exposure and subsequent analysis of images should be kept in mind (Table 7.1).

7.2.2 Choice of radioisotope

Although many radioisotopes (^{3}H, ^{14}C, ^{32}P, ^{33}P, ^{35}S and ^{125}I) have been used in ISH, a number of factors determine the suitability of different isotopes for a particular application. The anatomical resolution provided by an isotope is inversely related to the maximum energy of the β particles it emits (Rogers, 1979). Probes with low specific radioactivities and long half-lives (^{3}H and ^{14}C) provide excellent cellular resolution (e.g. Harlan et al. (1987) for ^{3}H), but require long exposure times, and for this reason are rarely used in ISH. One problem unique to ^{3}H is its differential self-absorption by tissues of different lipid content, leading to apparent variations in signal density where none exist. This problem is solved by defatting sections before exposing them to film or emulsion. ^{32}P-labelled probes, which emit β particles of very high energy, provide rapid results at the cost of cellular resolution, and may be used in situations where regional rather than cellular resolution is required. The short half-life of this isotope (14.3 days) gives it a very limited useful life. Probes labelled with ^{35}S and ^{33}P both provide good cellular resolution without requiring excessively long exposure times, and these are most commonly used in ISH. For these higher-energy isotopes, section thickness and the thickness of the emulsion layer are both critical in producing consistent results, as β particles emitted from the decay of these isotopes from the entire thickness of the section can produce a latent image on silver halide crystals throughout the extent of the emulsion layer (Rogers, 1979).

7.3 COMPUTERIZED IMAGE ANALYSIS SYSTEMS

The purpose of a computerized image analysis system (IAS) in the quantification of ISH is to convert experimental visual results into a format that can be processed to provide meaningful quantitative or semiquantitative information. A variety of approaches may be taken to achieve this objective, and this is reflected in the variety of IASs available to the researcher. With advances in digital technology and a greater understanding of the needs of bioscience research, modern IASs are faster, more powerful, easier to operate and substantially less expensive than

Table 7.1 Strategies to minimize variation in quantitative ISH results.

Procedure	Control
Obtaining tissue	Kill animals from different experimental groups at same time of day and in random order Identical dissection and freezing of tissues[a]

Cutting sections[b]	Cut sections from as many different groups as possible on to same microscope slide[c]
	 Position sections cut at the same anatomical level on the same slide[d]
	 Randomize or alternate order of cutting and mounting sections from different groups on slide, e.g.
	     slide series 1: animal group A, B, C
	     slide series 2: animal group B, C, A
	     slide series 3: animal group C, A, B[e]
	 (Consistent section thickness is critical)[f]

Section fixation, storage[g]	Fix all sections for a particular experiment at the same time and store together
Application of probe	Use the same batch of labelled probe for all sections to be analysed together[h]
Hybridization, washing	Perform at same time for all sections
Application to film, developing film	Co-expose all sections at the same time and for the same period (expose more than once if needed – see section 7.4.8 of text)[i] Position slides from each series throughout area of film (to minimize effects of variations in emulsion thickness) Only use X-ray cassettes that are in good condition (leaking or bent cassettes will result in uneven exposure or apposition of slides to film) Standardize film developing procedure[j]
Emulsion dipping development	Process all sections together using same batch of emulsion Standardize dipping procedure (temperature, time taken to dip each slide, drying)[k] Standardize emulsion development procedure

[a] For brain tissue, we use rapid removal of the brain at room temperature, followed by dissection in the coronal or sagittal plane with a single-edged razor blade. The brain is then rapidly frozen in a plastic weighing boat, with cut surface down, on (not in) liquid N_2. For dissection of the rat brain for sectioning in the flat skull position (corresponding to the atlas of Paxinos & Watson, 1986), we strongly recommend use of the Paxinos and Watson stereotaxic brain blocker (David Kopf Instruments, Tujunga, U.S.A.).

[b] We collect sections on to slides stored in the cryostat and thaw against the forefinger or the back of the hand. This allows section flattening and avoids wrinkling and folding of sections.

[c] For rat forebrain, three to four sections per slide is optimal; for rat medulla oblongata, up to ten sections may be placed on each slide. Sections should be positioned centrally on the slide to avoid uneven hybridization conditions near the edge of the parafilm coverslip and uneven emulsion thickness near the edge of the slide. If structures of interest (e.g. brain nuclei) are located laterally in the section, single hemispheres from control and experimental animals may be aligned before freezing and sectioning. This saves time and space, and gives directly comparable thickness of sections.

[d] When cutting rat brain, we monitor anatomical level using a low-power stereomicroscope with darkfield illumination base. While the section is still moist, anatomical details of white matter tracts versus grey-matter-enriched areas can be clearly identified and related to the acetylcholinesterase-stained sections of Paxinos & Watson (1986). While it is not essential to have closely matched anatomical levels on each slide, it makes analysis much more convenient and ensures that sections that are analysed together have been processed identically.

[e] This controls for the effects of exposure of the sections to different periods at room temperature or cryostat temperature before fixation or other pretreatments and storage before use.

[f] Uneven section thickness results in variable film optical density (OD) with higher-energy radioisotopes. Hence the usual precautions regarding the effectiveness of the cryostat/microtome should be adopted to ensure that the machine is not cutting 'thick–thin', shattered or wrinkled sections. Machines with fully adjustable mounting for tissue chucks allow more flexibility in collecting properly aligned sections.

[g] Post-sectioning fixation is optional under some new procedures (Dagerlind *et al.*, 1992; A.L. Gundlach, unpublished) but if tissue is to be fixed, time and conditions should be standardized. The ability to carry out ISH without any fixation may remove inconsistencies of fixation, particularly with perfusion-fixed animals, and may in fact give higher specific/background hybridization ratios.

(*notes h–k continued overleaf*)

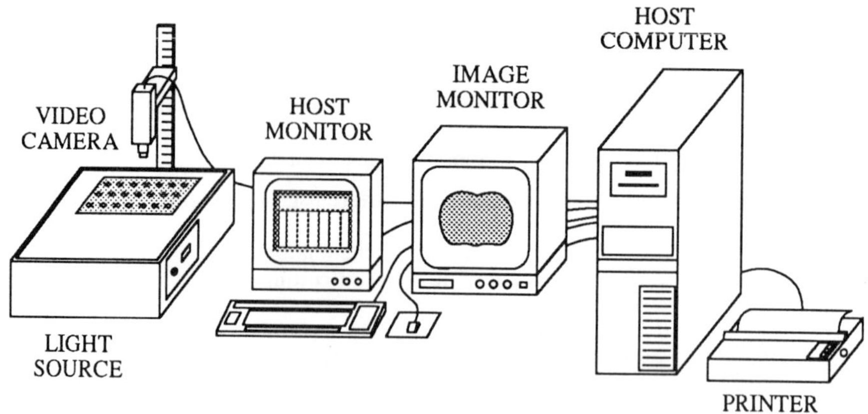

Figure 7.1 Basic components of a computerized image analysis system (see the text for details).

earlier systems, providing highly specialized procedures for rapid and accurate analysis of visual data. Whereas earlier systems were essentially custom built and programmed, many modern microcomputer-based IASs may be purchased complete ('off the shelf') or assembled around standard computer hardware.

The basic components of such a system, providing a means of image acquisition, processing, display, analysis, storage and output, are illustrated in Figure 7.1. The input device used depends on the type of visual data being analysed and the degree of detail required, and is generally a monochrome or colour video camera attached to a suitable lens or microscope. Specific types of input devices will be discussed in more detail in sections dealing with quantification of different types of ISH data.

Light intensities from the image are detected by the video camera as analogue electrical signals, which are then converted to digital format for processing by the computer. This digitization step breaks the image into discrete spatial elements (pixels), each of which has values for density (in grey levels) and specific X–Y location associated with it. Density is generally recorded with between 8 bits (corresponding to 256 grey levels) and 12 bits (4096 grey levels) of precision, and 256 × 256 to 2048 × 2048 pixels spatial resolution depending on the amount of space allocated to image memory. True colour systems generally assign 24 bits to colour, 8 bits each to red, green and blue. Greater memory space allows more detail to be obtained from images, but image memory is expensive, as are the more powerful processors required to manipulate these larger amounts of data. We find that 512 × 512 pixel × 256 grey level resolution is adequate for handling film images of ISH, and is also suitable for routine analysis of emulsion images.

In choosing an IAS, the researcher is faced with a range of options. Many modern systems are capable of analysing results from a variety of applications, and, in the absence of any specialist requirements, more than one system is likely to

---

(*Table 7.1 notes continued*)

[h] Labelling of probes to the same specific radioactivity is extremely difficult, so it is best to hybridize all experimental sections to be analysed for a single experiment with the same batch of probe or the same mixture of probes.

[i] There will be occasions when an increase or decrease in mRNA will mean that exposure time being optimized for control or treated sections will result in underexposure or saturation of some other images. Film or emulsion saturation (OD greater than 1.0 or silver grains overlying one another) seriously affects the accuracy of sampling, and should be avoided if at all possible (Davenport & Hall, 1988; Davenport & Nunez, 1990; Rogers, 1979).

[j] Many labs would use automated developing machines for Kodak X-Omat film (for instance we use a machine available 24 h a day in our hospital X-ray department). If Hyperfilm β-Max (or other films requiring separate development) is used, it is important to use the same recommended development temperature, time and chemicals on all occasions.

[k] This is necessary for obtaining emulsion layers of consistent thickness, which are vital for accurate quantification (see Section 7.5.3 of text). A potential problem with emulsion drying is that emulsion tends to run from the top to the bottom of the slide before drying. Avoid placing sections too close to the end of the microscope slide.

be suitable for the routine analysis of ISH results. Choice of systems must then be based on criteria other than just the ability to perform the necessary quantification of experimental results. It may be difficult for the researcher to meaningfully evaluate the performance of different IASs even if access to working systems is possible. Discussion with experienced users of different systems is invaluable, and may inform potential buyers of the ease of use as well as the advantages and shortcomings of particular systems. A study of the literature in an appropriate field of research may give some indication of which systems are commonly used, but will not necessarily reveal the best, most recent or most economical options.

The rapidity of change in computer technologies leads to continual refinements in hardware and software, so the ability to easily upgrade or update components of the IAS is a distinct advantage. Systems with modular design and software-update availability allow the researcher to keep pace with advances in image analysis technology, and lessen the risk of being left with obsolete equipment. Flexibility of hardware and software options within a given system also allows tailoring of the system to specific or multiple needs the user may have which were not present (or not envisaged) when the system was initially purchased, avoiding the expense of duplicating system components. Cost, or at least perceived value for money, is also likely to be an important consideration for most groups in selecting an IAS.

We use the microcomputer imaging device (MCID) M1 system from Imaging Research Inc. (St. Catharines, Ontario, Canada), which runs on an IBM compatible 80386 or 486 computer under the powerful OS/2 operating system. This system is of modular design, and includes integrated software modules for many bioscience applications, some of which will be discussed in later sections. Custom software for specialist applications may also be obtained from the supplier of this system. An advantage of microcomputer-based IASs is the ability to export data directly to spreadsheet and statistical packages (running on the same computer or another compatible machine) for further analysis, avoiding the time-consuming process of re-entering data for this purpose.

Different IASs use different methods of displaying images and other data. The MCID systems utilize two monitors: one to display measured data and interactions with the host computer (host monitor) and another to display images (image monitor; see Figure 7.1). Displayed images may be processed in a number of ways, and various types of image data can be recorded. As well as visual output, numerical data and images may be printed (using a suitable graphics printer or thermal transfer printer for images) or stored on disk or tape for later retrieval. Photographic prints or slides of images may be obtained by direct photography of the image monitor or by use of a film recorder (which produces images of slightly lower quality than direct photography).

While not essential for the quantification of film ISH, visual enhancement of images is useful in illustrating experimental observations as well as assisting in such processes as setting threshold densities during analysis. To our knowledge, all computerized IASs allow for pseudocolour coding of grey scale values. This feature simplifies the perception of differences in signal density, as the human eye can more readily distinguish differences in colour than in shades of grey (see Colour Plate 1).

7.4 QUANTIFICATION OF FILM IMAGES OF ISH

7.4.1 Introduction

The apposition of sections hybridized with radioactively labelled probes to X-ray film allows the rapid quantification of gene expression at the regional (but not cellular) level of brain and other tissues. The optical density (OD) of film images produced by these sections is related (though not necessarily in a linear manner) to the regional radioactivity concentration, and thus represents the relative amount of target mRNA present in the sections. In order to determine regional radioactivity values (and hence relative abundance of mRNA), experimental images must be compared with those produced by samples of known radioactive content which are co-exposed to film with the hybridized sections. The production of radioactive standards, the fitting of standard curves, and the sampling of experimental results (including extrapolation from standard curves) are all procedures that need to be understood in order to gain accurate and reproducible data. Some knowledge of the limitations of film-based autoradiography and its quantification is also important.

7.4.2 Resolution of film images

The degree of resolution (and hence the amount of anatomical information) that can be gained from film-based emulsions is limited in part by the emulsion type used. (Resolution is also influenced by the choice of radioisotope, section thickness, the closeness of apposition between the sections and film, and the length of exposure; these factors are discussed elsewhere in this chapter.) Different X-ray films are distinguished by the thickness and characteristics of their emulsion layer (the size of the silver halide crystals, the size of the developed silver grains and the sensitivity of the emulsion to β particles of different energies). All of these factors determine the suitability of the film to a particular application as well as the resolution which can be achieved using the film (see Rogers, 1979). Many currently available X-ray films are suitable for use in ISH, with the most commonly used being Kodak X-Omat and Amersham Hyperfilm β-Max. Kodak X-Omat is made with a high silver content emulsion on both sides of a clear plastic base, and produces images of reasonably good resolution from the shortest possible exposure time. Amersham Hyperfilm β-Max has a single sided emulsion of very high silver content which combines improved resolution with short exposure times and lower background. This film is more expensive than Kodak X-Omat and generally requires separate (manual) development – it cannot be processed in an automated X-ray film developer without adjustment of the development and fixation times. Other films, such as Agfa Curix Ortho ST-G2 and DuPont Cronex-4, may require longer exposure times, but can give lower background levels than

X-Omat and may be a more economical option (for example, we can obtain Agfa film from our hospital X-ray department at a very reasonable bulk rate).

7.4.3 System requirements for quantification of film images

For accurate quantification of film images of ISH, sources of variation in illumination and recording of films must be removed or their effects minimized. Most commonly, a video camera attached to a photographic lens is used to capture images of the film, which is illuminated from below. Any variation in camera performance or lighting conditions ultimately affects the accuracy of data recorded, so the use of optimal and standardized conditions for the digitization of images is essential for meaningful quantification. The major sources of error in image digitization conditions (variations in camera performance and in lighting parameters) may be controlled by careful selection of imaging components and attention to analysis conditions. The ability of the light source to produce stable illumination in the presence of variations in power supply and over sustained periods is critical for accurate measurement. A good IAS should allow for the correction of shading errors brought about by an uneven pattern of illumination or irregularities in camera performance (e.g. lower sensitivity at extremes compared with centre of field). These features, plus the uniformity of ambient lighting in the immediate environment around the IAS, assist the operator in obtaining accurate and reproducible results.

For analysis of film images, we use a Sony XC-77CE solid-state video camera with Canon television camera lens attached to a Nikon micro Nikkor 55 mm f 2.8 lens and Vivitar extension tube set (standard with our MCID M1 system). Coupled to a Kaiser RS1 copy stand, this configuration allows for a wide range of magnifications, appropriate for many different experimental situations (e.g. visualization of a whole rat brain section or analysis of detail in small brain nuclei). Film illumination is supplied by the Northern Light Precision Illuminator model B90 (also from Imaging Research Inc.), which provides constant lighting (the intensity of which can be set by the operator) with digital readout of lamp power, and is specified to exhibit less than 0.05% drift over 12 h. External light in the image analysis environment may be controlled by dim ambient lighting conditions, although we prefer to use opaque cardboard tubes surrounding the camera lens and extending down over the film to exclude room light.

7.4.4 System calibration

The performance of any computerized IAS depends on how well the system is prepared to carry out the quantification required. For obtaining reliable measures, a standard quantification procedure should be adhered to, with exact analysis conditions being optimized for the type of analysis being performed. The exact details of calibration depend on the system being used and the particular application, but the basic processes involved are described below.

7.4.4.1 *Set camera magnification and focus*

The camera position and focus must be set to provide appropriate magnification for the regions to be studied. It is obviously convenient to be able to digitize large regions in one step, so too high a magnification factor is to be avoided. For acceptable accuracy at the other extreme, magnification must be sufficient for regions to be at least 3 to 4 pixels wide (assuming 512×512 pixel image memory; Ramm, 1990). When targets of different sizes are to be analysed on a single film, it is more convenient if all sampling can be carried out at one magnification, even if different regions must be digitized separately.

7.4.4.2 *Spatial distance calibration*

If absolute distance or area measurements are to be recorded from film images, distance calibration must be performed each time the system magnification is altered. We use a good-quality transparent Perspex ruler placed under the video camera to define distances (in mm or μm), which are then used to convert the number of pixels to an absolute measure of distance or area. In the

absence of this calibration, the IAS can still record distances or areas in pixels, but these measurements are only relevant to the particular magnification conditions under which they are recorded.

7.4.4.3 *Shading error correction and lighting adjustment*

Shading error correction is a pixel by pixel adjustment process which is performed to compensate for variations in background density (shading) over the field of view. These variations are due to inconsistencies in the illumination pattern (from the light source and the imaging environment) and in camera and lens performance. Shading error correction needs to be carried out when the relationship of the imaging components changes (e.g. as a result of moving the light source or changing the magnification). Once this correction is performed, data may be sampled from multiple films as long as the imaging components are not moved relative to each other. For our system, shading error is corrected by digitizing a blank field with the lighting set so that the OD of this blank field is at the mid-range of values encountered in analysis.

Reading density data from regions at the extremes of the OD range must be avoided for accurate quantification of film images. Regulating exposure times can prevent saturation of film images (see Section 7.4.8), while correct adjustment of the illumination level for analysis avoids the problems of images being too bright. Optimal illumination levels may vary for different IASs, and, for analysis with MCID systems, it is recommended that lighting is adjusted to produce ODs of 0.05–0.1 for areas of film background.

7.4.4.4 *Standard curve fitting*

Film response to radioactive emissions is not linear, so a way of relating film OD to tissue radioactivity content is required. To achieve this, film images produced by a set of standards (see Protocol 7.1) of known radioactivity are analysed, and a calibration curve is interpolated from these standards to assign values to experimental samples between the points on this curve (see

Protocol 7.1 Preparation of ^{35}S-labelled brain paste standards.

Many investigators have adopted the use of isotope-impregnated tissue standards as a means of calibrating the IAS for quantitative analysis. While a large number of protocols exist for the preparation of these standards, most of these are essentially modifications of a similar procedure. We have found the following method to be simple and convenient and to provide reproducible results over many batches of radioactivity.

For the preparation of ten standards, which span a 1000-fold concentration range, we follow these steps.

1. Homogenize whole brain (or brain less cerebellum) from two rats with mortar and pestle. Place 100 μl (approx) aliquots in separate 1.5 ml microcentrifuge tubes, labelled 1 to 10. Centrifuge briefly (30 s) to remove air bubbles and pack down homogenate.
2. Prepare dilutions of radioactivity in distilled water (dH$_2$O). Add 1 μl of [α-^{35}S]dATP (specific radioactivity 12.5 Ci μl^{-1} or about 2.8 × 10^7 d.p.m. μl^{-1}) to 19 μl of dH$_2$O to make dilution 'A'. Count 1 μl (or convenient volume) of 'A' (should be about 1.4 × 10^6 d.p.m. μl^{-1}).
3. For 50 000 d.p.m. mg^{-1} wet weight brain tissue (or 5 million d.p.m. 100 mg^{-1}), you need (5 × 10^6) / (1.4 × 10^6) or 3.6 μl of 'A' in 100 mg of brain paste → standard 1.
4. For ten standards distributed over 1000-fold range (50–50 000 d.p.m. mg^{-1}), each successive dilution needs to be by a factor of 1000$^{1/9}$ or 1/2.15. So:
    Add 10 μl of 'A' to 11.5 μl of dH$_2$O → dilution 'B'.
    Then add 3.6 μl of 'B' to 100 mg of brain paste → standard 2.
    Repeat for dilutions 'C' to 'J' (standards 3–10).
5. Mix all standards well and centrifuge briefly. Repeat 'mix/centrifuge' step three times.
6. Count radioactivity from about 10 mg (record weights) of each brain paste standard to get d.p.m. mg^{-1} values. This is best carried out by adding tissue to preweighed scintillation vials, recording the final weight and solubilizing radioactivity with scintillant overnight before counting. (Some investigators prefer to count radioactivity from a number of sections, cut as in step 8 below, either weighing the sections or simply recording an average amount of radioactivity for sections of each standard which can be related to the area of the section during system calibration).
7. Mix again, centrifuge and freeze standards.
8. Cut sections of desired thickness (same as thickness to be used for experimental tissues). Two standards can be conveniently mounted on the chuck at the same time and cut concurrently. To remove frozen standard blocks from microcentrifuge tubes for cutting, cut a small piece from the bottom of the tube and carefully shake or push block out.

An alternative to the use of microcentrifuge tubes for the preparation of brain paste standards is to use 1 ml disposable plastic syringes, giving standards of identical diameter which may be removed by cutting off the tip of the syringe and squeezing out the frozen standard blocks.

Colour Plate 1). Owing to slight differences in film apposition and between-film variation in silver content (however small these factors may be), it is good practice to co-expose radioactive standards with every sheet of film and to create a standard curve for each film exposure. Each standard may then be digitized, and OD ($\pm$ area; Protocol 7.1) recorded. Once this is done for all standards over an appropriate range for the film, a curve is fitted to the density values (calibrated in appropriate units; Protocol 7.1). A number of curve types have been used to fit radioactivity standards, with log–log plots most commonly used. The 'best' curve type to use with a given set of standards and exposure conditions is the one that provides the most accurate fit to the points, and IASs generally provide a range of mathematical functions from which to choose. It is not necessary to always use the same curve type as different exposure conditions and different sets of standards can produce different responses.

It is possible to record uncalibrated OD measurements (i.e. without reference to a standard curve), to ascertain whether one target is darker or lighter than another. This procedure is, however, critically dependent on the lighting conditions used, and values recorded in this way have no fixed reference point.

The use of radioisotopes with a relatively short half-life (e.g. ^{33}P, ^{35}S) necessitates the preparation of new standards on a regular basis to ensure that standards produce a range of OD values that is appropriate for comparison with experimental samples. One strategy for avoiding this procedure is to cross-calibrate standards of the isotope used in ISH with standards of an isotope that emits β particles of similar energy but that has a longer half-life. ^{14}C fulfils these criteria, and standards incorporating this isotope may be purchased or prepared using any stable ^{14}C-labelled compound and a procedure similar to that of Protocol 7.1. A conversion factor, relating the film OD produced by the two radioisotopes, may be determined from co-exposure of both sets of standards to film. In subsequent studies, ^{14}C standards alone may be co-exposed with ISH slides and the conversion factor used to relate film OD to tissue concentration of the isotope used to label ISH probes.

The actual units of radioactivity used to create standard curves are not critical, and there are many ways of describing the same values. While we normally prepare our standards and calibrate the IAS in d.p.m. mg^{-1} wet weight, units such as nCi mg^{-1} of protein or fmol µm^{-2} are equally valid.

7.4.5 Sampling of film images

IASs generally provide a choice of sampling methods for the quantification of film images. These sampling methods range from manual (where the user traces the outline of areas of interest) to fully automated (where all areas darker than a particular threshold OD or grey scale value are analysed), with the choice of method being dependent on such factors as the type of targets being studied (e.g. discrete nuclei versus a relatively homogeneous pattern of distribution) and the type of numerical data required (e.g. density, area, number of discrete targets). A study of the literature dealing with ISH reveals no consensus of sampling methods or reported data, as individual researchers or groups have adopted their own standard quantification procedures. It is obvious that no single method will work well for every application, and in deciding which method(s) to use the twin objectives of accuracy and reproducibility must be foremost in mind. The most common sampling methods, and some of their potential applications, are discussed below.

7.4.5.1 Manual outlining

This is the most time-consuming method of sampling data, and may also be subject to the greatest operator bias and between-operator variations in sampling (e.g. see Eilbert *et al.*, 1990). For some applications this method may still be the most suitable or the only method available, although more recent image analysis software tends to provide faster and more reproducible alternatives. In its favour, manual sampling allows the skilled operator to define and analyse complex shapes or nuclei which vary dramatically in shape and size at different anatomical levels (which are thus difficult to outline using templates). Density and area of

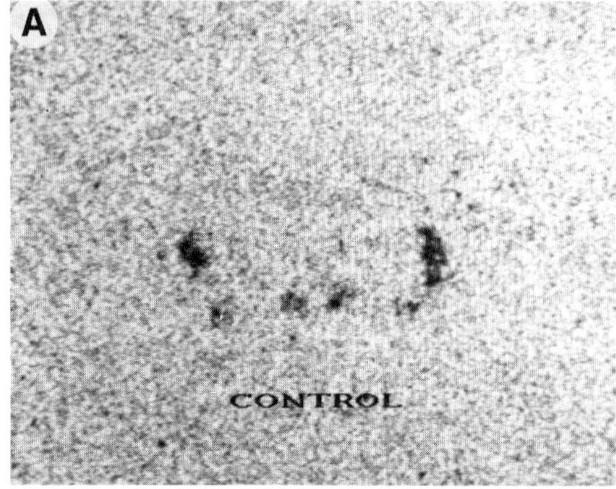

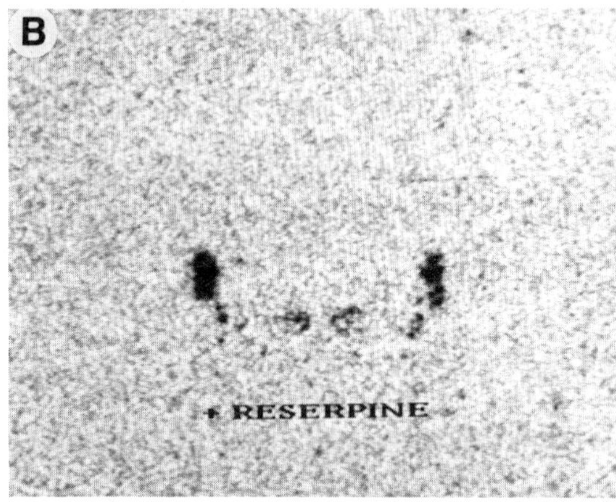

Figure 7.2 X-ray film images of pre-proneuropeptide Y mRNA distribution in locus coeruleus from (A) control and (B) reserpine-treated (10 mg kg^{-1}, intra-peritoneal, 24 h) rats. Midline structures indicate the presence of this mRNA in dorsal tegmental nuclei. Computerized image analysis of multiple sections from three animals per group revealed an increase of 145 ± 12% in locus coeruleus mRNA abundance after reserpine treatment.

hybridization recorded using this method may both provide meaningful data. An example of manual outlining is shown in Colour Plate 1(E). Using this sampling method, and recording calibrated density values without area measurement from a series of film images such as those in Figure 7.2, we detected a 145% increase in the abundance of pre-proneuropeptide Y mRNA in the locus coeruleus of the rat 24 h after reserpine treatment (10 mg kg^{-1} intraperitoneal administration).

7.4.5.2 Geometric sampling tools

Most IASs provide a number of these tools, which the user may alter in size and orientation. The operator then simply positions the shape over the regions of interest to record signal density and other data. This method is relatively fast, and allows areas of identical size and shape, of appropriate dimensions for the regions being investigated, to be sampled from multiple sections or samples. Some operator decision is required in the choice of size and shape of the sampling window and in its placement, but consistency of analysis may be achieved by always positioning the window in the same way, e.g. over the most lateral aspect of a nucleus or the area of densest signal. This method of sampling is only useful in recording density data, and so would not be appropriate in situations where the size of the target under study is subject to variation due to experimental treatments, for instance if cells from a larger area express a particular gene following treatment or in developmental studies.

7.4.5.3 User-defined templates

User-defined templates are used in the same way as the geometric sampling tools, and may be saved and recalled for later use. These templates allow consistent sampling of density values from regions of interest which are not accurately defined by geometric sampling tools.

7.4.5.4 Automatic sampling

Using automatic sampling methods, outlines are created by the image analysis software using OD or grey scale thresholds to distinguish targets from background areas. The operator must define a sample window (by selecting the whole of a section or only some part of it) and select the threshold level. This threshold may be fixed for the sampling of all areas or may be varied by the operator to compensate for changes in background hybridization signal. Determination of the threshold level introduces the possibility of inappropriate sampling for some targets if the threshold level is fixed at a particular OD or grey scale level, or of operator bias or inconsistency when variable thresholds are used. Care must also be taken to accurately and consistently define an appropriate sampling window. Automatic sampling may be of use when regions of study are of variable size, but is difficult to perform when targets are poorly distinguishable from background. Selection of appropriate threshold levels is critical for accurate and reproducible automatic sampling, as small changes in threshold values may lead to larger variations in average density or target area. An example of automatic sampling of density and area data is shown in Colour Plate 1(F).

7.4.5.5 *Other sampling strategies*

Whichever of the above (or other) sampling methods are used, the operator must also decide how to distinguish regions of interest from background and record specific hybridization signals. The techniques of redirected sampling and image subtraction are common to many modern IASs, and deserve some attention at this point.

Using *redirected sampling*, multiple images may be overlaid and stored in different channels or different image memory areas. Redirected sampling may be used to define regions of interest (using histological identification by appropriate staining of sections) or to define non-specific hybridization (using consecutive sections to those showing 'total' hybridization). In the first of these cases, the autoradiographic image of hybridization signal is digitized in one channel, and a corresponding section, stained with a histochemical or biochemical marker to identify regions of interest, is aligned with the first and stored in another channel, linked to the original one. Targets are defined from the histology (using outlining or geometric sampling tools), and data are read from the corresponding area of the autoradiograph. In this way, data may be obtained from nuclei which are not easily identified by their hybridization pattern alone. Another possibility, or an extension of the above method, is to digitize an aligned image of non-specific hybridization into an additional channel, so that values of total and non-specific hybridization may be recorded from the two channels simultaneously. This may be considered an expensive alternative as large amounts of cold oligonucleotide probe are needed to generate images of non-specific hybridization. The issue of controls for specific hybridization is discussed further in Section 7.4.7.

Redirected sampling can reduce uncertainty in defining regions of interest and assist in sampling appropriate areas from multiple sections simultaneously. If redirected sampling is not available on the IAS being used, it may be possible to simulate this feature. Outlines may be drawn to highlight areas of interest on a digitized image of a stained section, and then, while retaining the overlaid outlines, other sections may be digitized and aligned with these outlines and data sampled from the appropriate areas.

Image subtraction is another tool commonly (but perhaps not always appropriately) used in quantifying autoradiographs. In this operational mode, two calibrated images may be aligned, and the hybridization signal from one (non-specific hybridization, for instance) may be digitally subtracted from the other (total hybridization) to produce a digital image of specific signal with grey scales determined from reference to the standard curve. This technique is useful for illustrating specific hybridization (e.g. for publication or other display), which may appear quite different from total signal. In our opinion, however, image subtraction should not be used for the quantification of specific hybridization for two reasons. Firstly, it is extremely difficult to align two images perfectly, even using the sophisticated alignment algorithms available in some IASs. Often even serial or near-adjacent sections appear slightly different when placed on slides. Imperfect alignment leads to a reduction in the accuracy of quantification. In addition, the image-subtraction procedure is subject to round-off errors, which become more of a problem at the extremes of the calibration scale.

7.4.6 Recording of image data

The type of data recorded from film images of hybridization is to a large extent dependent on the sampling method used, so sampling should be tailored to the particular application to provide accurate regional measurements or to reveal changes between experimental groups. If cells from a larger area are recruited to express a particular gene following experimental treatments, as is often the case, then it is important to document the area of hybridization signal associated with the regions of interest. In this case, fixed-size sampling tools are inappropriate, and manual or computerized outlining of targets is necessary. Alternatively, or in addition, the average hybridization density may be altered due to changes in the average number of copies of the target mRNA per cell, so under these circumstances density values must be noted to determine the magnitude of any changes seen. Some researchers prefer to report the area $\times$ density product, as this presumably reflects the total amount of mRNA present and takes into account changes in both determinants. It is up to the individual researcher to ensure that the analytical techniques used enable the reliable detection of a change in gene expression in their experimental paradigm if and only if such a change exists.

7.4.7 Controls for use with film autoradiography

A number of procedures may be used to assess the specificity of ISH results (Chapter 1). When working with a new oligonucleotide, the researcher should check that the radiolabelled probe is displaced by an excess (10- to 100-fold) of unlabelled probe. A sense probe, equivalent in length and G-C content to the oligonucleotide being used, is also useful in evaluating the authentic nature of hybridization with the antisense probe by measuring non-specific hybridization levels. For routine analysis using a familiar probe, these rigid controls are not necessary. We generally recognize specific hybridization as that above the section background signal (which may be due to such factors as chemography, non-specific adhesion of probe or hybridization of tailed probes to poly(T) regions in cells). This level of background should be uniformly low in all sections, and be equivalent to that seen in the presence of an excess of unlabelled probe. Generally, if hybridization has been carried out correctly, regions known not to express the gene being studied have density readings only slightly above film background levels, and signal from

these regions is used to define section background, which is subtracted from all readings to give values for specific hybridization.

7.4.8 Film exposure times

Films used in ISH approach saturation at an OD of approximately 1.0; above this limit, increases in radioactivity produce little or no further increase in labelling density (see Colour Plate 1 and also Davenport & Hall, 1988; Davenport & Nunez, 1990). For accurate quantification, it is important to control film exposure times to prevent saturation of film over regions of interest. If this practice is not observed, changes in the abundance of target mRNA may be underestimated or even not perceived. Images that are too pale may be difficult to distinguish from film background, so multiple exposures may be necessary to quantify areas of widely differing densities, although this is seldom necessary in practice. Regions that are to be directly compared (i.e. the same region in different animals or multiple regions within animals) should be analysed from a single exposure time (preferably on the same sheet of film) if at all possible.

7.5 QUANTIFICATION OF NUCLEAR EMULSION IMAGES OF ISH

7.5.1 Introduction

The study of gene expression at the cellular level, using ISH combined with nuclear emulsion autoradiographic techniques, provides greater anatomical detail than film-based methods. The preparation and analysis of emulsion images of mRNA levels is, however, more technically complex and time-consuming than X-ray film methods. Whereas some researchers regularly analyse emulsion autoradiographs of ISH to provide quantitative information about gene expression, we prefer to use X-ray films for routine quantification and reserve the use of nuclear emulsions to provide qualitative detail of gene expression at a finer anatomical level. In some experimental situations, for instance if the mRNA of interest is only expressed in a small number of scattered neurons or is of low abundance, the regional distribution of mRNA is of little relevance, making emulsion autoradiography of hybridized sections a more suitable analytical method. Emulsion autoradiography is also useful in a variety of double-labelling situations; analysis of isotopic ISH may be carried out in conjunction with non-isotopic ISH, with immunocytochemistry or with conventional histological staining.

7.5.2 Theoretical aspects of quantifying emulsion images of ISH

ISH combined with emulsion autoradiography allows the study of the radioactivity concentration of single cells, and thus can provide information about the number of cells expressing the target mRNA as well as the relative level of expression within individual cells. As is the case for ISH combined with film autoradiography, the number of developed silver grains in the emulsion overlying single cells, within defined limits, is related to the radioactivity concentration (and hence the relative abundance of the target mRNA) in these cells.

While it may be tempting to use emulsion-coated radioactivity standards to produce a standard curve for analysis of emulsion images, and thus calibrate grain densities with known amounts of radioactivity (as for the analysis of film images), this technique is probably best avoided. Radioactivity sources of different shapes and sizes affect emulsions differently (Rogers, 1979), so it cannot be assumed that a homogeneous source of radioactivity (such as a tissue or plastic standard) will produce the same grain density as a smaller source (e.g. a cell) containing the same concentration of radioactivity. For this reason, it is necessary to determine directly the density of developed silver grains in the emulsion over areas of the tissue under investigation, and to use these grain density values as the relative measures of radioactivity content (and hence of target gene expression).

The relationship between the radioactivity concentration of tissue and the density of grains over this tissue is not linear but logarithmic (i.e. the number of β particles entering the emulsion increases more rapidly than does its grain density), although the first part of this logarithmic curve is approximately linear (Rogers, 1979). Thus, up to a limiting grain density, the relative radioactivity concentration of different samples may be inferred from the density of developed silver grains in the emulsion over the samples, and meaningful comparisons between identically produced samples may be made. The limit of this linearity is related to the size of the undeveloped silver halide crystals in the emulsion, and is reached when some 10% of available crystals have been hit by β particles (Rogers, 1979). Although this theoretical limit may be difficult to determine in practice, the researcher should be aware that, apart from making precise grain-counting difficult, significant overlap (or even fusion) of developed grains may severely affect the accuracy of results obtained. From our experience, counts above some 100 grains per neuron become difficult to measure. Careful monitoring of emulsion exposure, by developing test slides at regular intervals, should be carried out to prevent saturation of the emulsion over the most heavily labelled cells, making analysis of images both easier and more accurate.

In the analysis of emulsion images of ISH, the two questions most commonly being addressed are: how many (or what proportion of) cells express the mRNA of interest (i.e. the number or proportion of radioactively labelled cells), and what is the average relative amount of this mRNA per labelled cell? While it may seem trivial, a problem exists in defining what constitutes a labelled or unlabelled cell. Areas of emulsion over cells which do not produce the mRNA of interest, and indeed over regions of non-neuronal tissue (such as myelin fibre tracts in brain and spinal cord), generally contain low levels of developed silver grains. As cells that express the target mRNA do so in varying amounts, the frequency distribution of grains per cell (or per unit area) over labelled cells may overlap with the distribution of grain density over unlabelled regions, if the target mRNA is of low abundance. Although complex formulae exist for estimating the proportion of labelled cells (e.g.

see Rogers, 1979), simpler methods can also give valid results. One relatively simple formula that may be used to distinguish labelled from unlabelled cells is to set a threshold grain density equal to or greater than that over 95% of cells known not to express the mRNA in question (e.g. see Burton *et al.*, 1992); any cell that has a grain density greater than this limit may then be assumed to be labelled and hence to produce the target mRNA. As is the case with X-ray film, background hybridization, in the form of (hopefully) low densities of silver grains, should be determined separately and subtracted from total grain density (i.e. specific plus background) before the statistical comparison of different samples. For the sake of accuracy, it is preferable that background be kept to a minimum, and attention should be paid to conditions used in the preparation, exposure and development of emulsions to minimize background.

7.5.3 Isotopes and emulsions

The anatomical resolution that can be achieved using nuclear emulsions is dependent on the isotope and emulsion used, as well as factors such as the section thickness, the length of exposure and the development conditions. As the radioisotopes most commonly used in ISH (^{35}S, ^{33}P) emit β particles which have path lengths greater than the emulsion thickness normally achieved (typically 3–4 μm (Rogers, 1979) using standard dipping procedures (Chapter 1)), the thickness of the emulsion layer is critical for obtaining reproducible results. Standardized procedures for the dipping, drying and development of emulsions are thus essential when these high-energy isotopes are utilized. The issue of consistent emulsion thickness is not critical when tritium-labelled probes are used, as the β particles from ^{3}H are very unlikely to travel more than 2 μm into the emulsion layer (Rogers, 1979). Differential self-absorption of this isotope by tissue regions of differing density, as well as the long exposure times needed to produce a suitable image, reduce the usefulness of tritium in emulsion ISH. Probes labelled with ^{32}P emit β particles of sufficiently high energies to cause the production of exposed silver grains at a

distance from their source, so the resolution that can be achieved using this isotope is unacceptable for the study of gene expression at the cellular level.

The characteristics of the particular nuclear emulsion used, including its grain density, grain size and sensitivity to β particles of different energies, are also important in determining the resolution which can be achieved. Several photographic supply companies market nuclear emulsions suitable for light microscopic analysis. The emulsions most commonly used in the study of ISH are Kodak NTB 2, Ilford K5 and Amersham LM1, which all have undeveloped grain diameters of between 0.20 and 0.26 μm. These emulsions do not require overly long exposure times, and can be diluted with water to adjust the emulsion concentration and thickness. We and others routinely use Ilford K5 emulsion, diluted 1:1 with water/1% glycerol as this gives a uniform emulsion layer of appropriate consistency (see Chapter 1, Protocol 1.9). This method is also convenient and more economical than using undiluted emulsion. Amersham LM1 and Kodak NTB 2 may give slightly quicker results than the Ilford material, but may not be suitable in cases where chemographic artefacts are observed in the presence of some tissue or reagent components (e.g. Trembleau *et al.*, 1993).

7.5.4 System requirements for quantification of emulsion images

A variety of techniques is available for the quantitative analysis of emulsion images of ISH, making any attempt to summarize or compare the different methods, as well as the exact equipment needed to perform them, extremely difficult. Grain counting may be performed manually, in which case only a microscope that allows suitable magnification for the visualization of individual grains is required. Far more commonly, however, this task is performed with the aid of a computerized IAS. For researchers who already have a microscope and IAS, the decision of which techniques to use may be based on the capabilities of their system, while for those just starting out in the field the number of options may be somewhat bewildering.

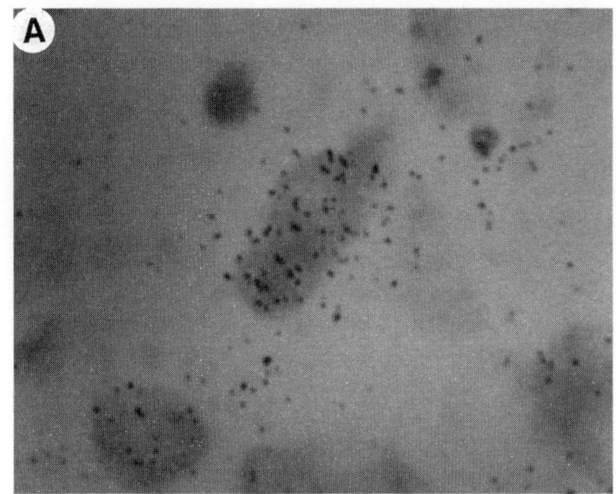

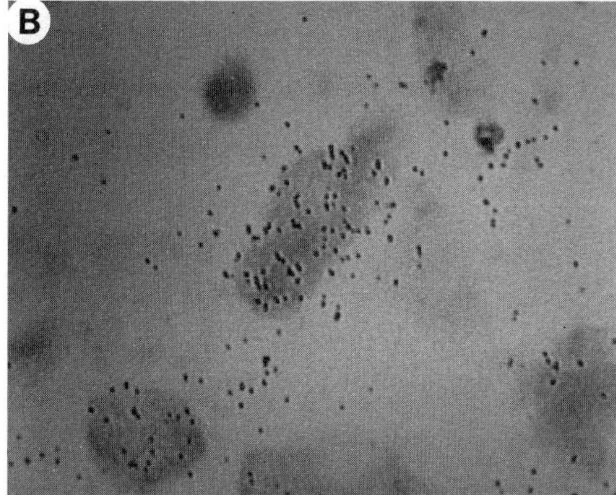

Figure 7.3 Emulsion autoradiographic images showing lateral hypothalamic cells expressing somatostatin mRNA. (A) Original image using 100× objective and oil immersion. Note low contrast between silver grains and stained cells, as well as some overlap of grains. (B) Field from (A) after image enhancement algorithm to highlight small dark objects. Grains are now clearly distinguishable from background.

The basic equipment needed to quantify ISH at the cellular level comprises a microscope coupled to an IAS. Many of the features of an IAS that are necessary for quantification of emulsion images are identical with those used for analysis of X-ray film images, which are discussed in Sections 7.3 and 7.4.3 (above). The ability to digitally enhance images (to increase the contrast between grains and underlying stained tissue – see Section 7.5.5.1 below and Figure 7.3) is an obvious advantage, as is the availability of automated grain-counting procedures. Both these features are common to modern IASs. As

is the case for the analysis of film images, facilities for the correction of shading errors also aid the accurate quantification of cellular mRNA. Some IASs feature motor stage tracking as an option, allowing the movement of the viewing stage in standard predetermined steps as well as permitting identical areas to be scanned under brightfield (BF) and later under darkfield (DF) conditions (or at different magnifications) without the need to constantly readjust the system when switching between the two viewing modes. The usefulness of the motor stage for some applications must, however, be weighed up against its relatively high cost.

For the quantification of ISH at the cellular level, attention to constant and standardized analysis conditions is crucial. Typically a light microscope is attached to the video camera of the IAS using a video adaptor. Many microscope light sources, for either BF or DF viewing, produce more variation in illumination than the light sources used for analysis of film images. This problem can be overcome to some extent by the use of a line voltage stabilizer. Most standard light microscopes which have an adjustable light source would be suitable for analysing emulsion autoradiographs of ISH. The ability to view slides under BF and DF conditions and to use a range of objectives to properly visualize silver grains in the emulsion layer are clear advantages. It is important that all components of the visual system (microscope and camera) are clean, as dust or other marks on any of these surfaces can obscure or distort object detail.

We use an Olympus BH-2 microscope fitted with objectives from 1× to 100× and with interchangeable BF and DF condensors. This microscope is coupled via an adaptor to the video camera of the MCID M1 system (described in Section 7.4.3). This system features grain counting (as well as grain area and proportional target area measurement), a range of image-enhancement functions which may be further customized by the operator, shading error correction and the ability to perform motor stage tracking (although we do not use this feature). The M1 system also allows flexible options for the handling of the data produced during analysis.

7.5.5 Sampling of emulsion images

The aim of analysis of emulsion images is to measure the abundance of developed silver grains over cells of interest, so sampling procedures must distinguish these grains from the underlying tissue. This is achieved using selection criteria (normally based on the size and darkness of grains) to highlight grains, which may then be counted or their area measured. In order to distinguish grains from counterstained cells, procedures involving image enhancement or viewing under DF conditions are generally used. The basic sampling procedures using these techniques are described below, and are also generally outlined in the operations manual of the IAS.

Although the size of individual silver grains in the emulsion layer will vary, the average grain size should be the same for all sections processed and developed identically using one batch of emulsion. For this reason, the area above a correctly chosen threshold density value (i.e. hybridization area) can accurately reflect the number of grains counted manually over a range of grain densities (Rogers *et al.*, 1987; Weiss & Chesselet, 1989; Smolen & Beaston-Wimmer, 1990), and has the advantage of avoiding the uncertainty in discerning individual grains when some overlap or fusion occurs. In order to use measurement of the area occupied by grains, the researcher should determine the limits between which a linear relationship between grain number and grain area exists. These limits will depend on factors such as the magnification used, the resolving power of the IAS, and the type of emulsion used. Manual grain counts and computerized area measurements (pixels or calibrated area) from cells with a wide range of grain densities should be used to construct a calibration curve relating grain number to grain area. Linear regression analysis may be used to determine a line of best fit, the slope of which is then used as a conversion factor to relate grain density to area above threshold for all cells from a particular experiment. Under a range of analysis conditions, a linear relationship between grain density and grain area has been demonstrated for from 10 to 150 grains per cell (Rogers *et al.*, 1987; Weiss & Chesselet, 1989; Smolen & Beaston-Wimmer, 1990).

7.5.5.1 Emulsion autoradiograph analysis under BF illumination

Under BF conditions, developed silver grains appear as black specks above the stained tissue. Critical to the analysis of emulsion images under these conditions is reliably distinguishing grains from the underlying tissue. Light counterstaining of cells, so that cell detail is only just visible, aids in this endeavour. Image-enhancement operations, which are a feature of most IASs, also greatly increase the contrast between cells and grains. These procedures modify images by changing the intensity value of each pixel, basing the new value on those of the surrounding pixels. In the case of grain counting, small dark objects (grains) are highlighted relative to larger pale objects (cells) using target accentuation or sharpening filters (see Figure 7.3 for an example). More sophisticated image enhancement, discriminating targets by their size and shape, may be used to separate contiguous targets (e.g. overlaid silver grains) before counting. Image processing operations do, by their nature, change image data, so the researcher should ensure that any processing operations carried out do not bias results in a way that will alter the outcome of a study.

An example of the analysis of emulsion images under BF viewing conditions is given in Protocol 7.2.

7.5.5.2 Emulsion autoradiograph analysis under DF illumination

The use of DF illumination to quantify emulsion images of ISH provides greater contrast between developed silver grains and stained tissue, and may avoid the need to use image processing routines to distinguish grains. Under these conditions, bright clear silver grains are visible over a dark background, with cells faintly visible due to their counterstaining. Lewis *et al.* (1989) found that more reliable quantification could be achieved with DF conditions than using the same magnification under BF illumination. One disadvantage of DF viewing is that slides and sections must be thoroughly clean to avoid artefacts caused by dust and other contaminants.

Analysis of emulsions under DF illumination is carried out in a manner almost identical with that described in Protocol 7.2 for BF, with the

Protocol 7.2 Steps in the analysis of emulsion autoradiographs under BF conditions.

1. Select magnification and adjust condensor. We find that, using 40× to 100× objective lenses (with oil immersion for 100×), individual grains may be distinguished, and the relative density of grains over different regions may be compared. Higher magnifications allow greater numerical accuracy by increasing the pixel/grain ratio, but slow down analysis by necessitating frequent movement of the viewing field. Check that the viewing field is of appropriate size for the tissue under investigation, and focus the microscope on the emulsion layer. Condensor aperture and height should be appropriate for the objective being used (see operations manual for microscope).
2. Shading error correction, to remove non-uniform illumination conditions over the field of view (see Section 7.4.4.3), should be carried out without a slide present, after the microscope has been focused.
3. Find an appropriate field of view to quantify. The researcher should decide (preferably before the start of sampling) which (and how many) cells to quantify in order to gain meaningful and representative data. The abundance and distribution of the target mRNA species, as well as the number of sections or animals available for study, will obviously influence the number and type of cells from different regions which can be sampled. It is important to have clear goals in mind before sampling in order to ensure that sufficient and appropriate data are obtained. As cells in each section will be transected at different levels and hence will have widely differing cross-sectional areas, it may be advisable to adopt some standard inclusion and exclusion criteria, for example only sampling from cells that have the nucleus in view.
4. Check focus each time the field of view is adjusted, to ensure that most grains are sharp. At high magnification, some grains will appear out of focus, but this is unavoidable.
5. Digitize image and perform image-enhancement procedures (where necessary) to increase contrast (Figure 7.3).
6. Set OD threshold for analysis. After image enhancement, grains should be easily distinguishable from the underlying tissue. Threshold is adjusted so that grains are selected while underlying tissue is not. It is our view, and has been verified by others (e.g. Lewis *et al.*, 1989), that adjusting the threshold for each cell or field of view, rather than using the same threshold value for all measurements, compensates for variations in lighting and in the staining density of underlying tissue, and so gives more reproducible results.
7. Define the region(s) to be sampled. The drawing and geometric tools described in Section 7.4.5 may be used to select areas of the field to be analysed. With ^{35}S and isotopes of similar energy, some scatter of silver grains around the actual cell is observed, so a standard method of defining target areas must be devised. One example would be to draw a border at a set distance outside the cell boundary for each cell to be analysed.
8. Sample from a defined area. Automated grain or pixel counting procedures give a value for the number of grains or pixels above threshold. As the size of cells may change as a result of some experimental treatments, grain or pixel *density*, rather than just number, is a more reliable measure of mRNA abundance, and requires the recording of the area sampled as well as the grain or pixel count for the area. Thus, for each sampling region, the number of grains per unit area or the proportion of the total sampling area above threshold (area above threshold/total area) may be recorded.
9. Sample next area (repeat steps 1–8).

exception that bright rather than dark targets are selected by thresholding. As is the case for BF viewing, a highly significant correlation between manually counted grains and computer-generated pixel counts may be achieved with DF illumination (Rogers *et al.*, 1987).

7.5.5.3 *Reflectance measurement under DF illumination*

If the developed emulsion layer is illuminated by a narrow beam of light directed downward through the objective lens, the amount of light reflected by the silver grains in the emulsion is directly proportional to grain density once system background is subtracted (see Rogers, 1979). Using a commercially available vertical incident illuminator, and viewing sections at relatively low magnifications, reflectance measurements of emulsion images may thus be obtained. The calibration of these reflectance measurements to the actual grain number is somewhat tedious, as the number of grains over single cells (viewed at high magnification) must be correlated with the reflectance of the same cells at lower power. For accuracy, readings from a large number of cells should be used for this calibration. After calibration, measures of number of labelled cells and average reflectance per cell (correlated with grain density) may be recorded from large areas of tissue quite rapidly.

Using this method of quantification, the stability of the light source is critical, as changes in lighting intensity will affect the reflectance measurements obtained. In addition, the amount of light reflected by silver grains is increased with increasing development time (Rogers, 1979), making standard and reproducible development of emulsions of vital importance. Owing to these technical limitations, as well as the ease and accuracy of other analysis methods, reflected light measurement is only rarely used in the quantification of nuclear emulsion autoradiographs of ISH.

7.5.6 **Controls for use with emulsion autoradiography**

As well as employing control strategies to assess the specificity of hybridization (Chapter 1 and Section 7.4.7), the researcher should also follow a number of procedures to ensure the validity of results obtained from the emulsion autoradiographic techniques used (Rogers, 1979). Silver grains may be produced in the emulsion by a number of sources other than the radioactively labelled probe which is hybridized to sections, so false positive results should be controlled for by the emulsion dipping and development of non-radioactive (i.e. non-hybridized) sections along with every batch of experimental slides. In addition, silver grains may be lost from areas of specific hybridization (i.e. false negative results). To control for this occurrence, a hybridized slide may be exposed to light at the time of dipping and then exposed and processed with experimental slides. Any loss of emulsion response over the hybridized tissue indicates (most commonly) chemography or fading of the latent image during exposure (Rogers, 1979), factors that could seriously affect the accuracy of quantifying other sections.

7.6 QUANTIFICATION OF NON-ISOTOPIC ISH

A relatively recent innovation in the study of gene expression is the use of non-isotopic ISH methods. These techniques offer improved (cellular and regional) resolution and faster results when compared with conventional radioactive methods, and dispense with the need for safety procedures which must be observed when radioactivity is used. The use of these techniques in quantitative ISH is not yet widespread, although their popularity is growing as better and simpler methods are devised.

Non-isotopic ISH methods involve either labelling of the probe (oligonucleotide, cDNA or cRNA) with a marker such as digoxigenin or biotin by the incorporation of a modified nucleotide, or the use of enzymes (alkaline phosphatase (AP) or horseradish peroxidase) which are conjugated to oligonucleotide probes by a 'linker arm' molecule during synthesis (Jablonski *et al.*, 1986; Emson, 1993). The reporter molecules are then utilized to produce a coloured or fluorescent reaction product, the abundance of which may be analysed quantitatively (see Augood *et al.*, 1992; Emson, 1993; Chapter 8).

In using non-isotopic methods in ISH, the same types of procedures as those used in conventional ISH (Table 7.1) should be observed to minimize the variability of results. As each step involved in the processing of sections and the amplification of signal introduces more chance of variability, the use of simpler procedures, such as those utilizing AP-labelled oligonucleotide probes (Augood *et al.*, 1992) may give more reproducible results.

Sections processed for non-isotopic ISH may be used to gain information about the number (or proportion) of cells expressing the target mRNA as well as the average relative level of labelling of these cells. Briefly, a microscope set to an appropriate magnification and coupled to a computerized IAS may be used to analyse labelled cells in a manner similar to that used for the study of emulsion images of ISH (Section 7.5, above). If cellular OD measurements are to be recorded, colour development should be carefully monitored to ensure that overdevelopment (analogous to film or emulsion saturation in isotopic ISH) does not occur. As no external standards are used in these procedures, it may not be appropriate to compare data across experiments. Sections from individual experiments may be compared with each other, and changes in the number of positive cells or the degree of labelling may be seen after experimental treatments (Augood *et al.*, 1992).

Non-isotopic ISH may also be used to study gene expression at the regional level, using analysis techniques akin to those used for film images (Section 7.4, above). Once again, the absence of external standards limits the validity of comparisons made across experiments using this method.

7.7 STATISTICAL ANALYSIS AND REPORTING OF RESULTS

The intelligent and appropriate statistical analysis of results from ISH and the ability to accurately describe these findings are important and often overlooked aspects of the study of gene expression using this technique. As more researchers (and referees!) gain expertise in statistical methods, the 'one test fits all' mentality in molecular biosciences is gradually being replaced by the economical use of appropriate statistical tests. A detailed description of statistical methods is beyond the scope of this article, and the reader is advised to refer to any of the many appropriate texts on biostatistics and analysis (e.g. Sokal & Rohlf, 1981; Armitage & Berry, 1987).

7.7.1 Some notes on statistics in the quantification of ISH

There is seldom consensus between authors on the exact methods of statistical analysis that are appropriate for their experimental results, and this state reflects both the broad array of possibilities and the absence (in most cases) of a single 'best' solution. Many different statistical software packages are available to the researcher, and the capabilities of the programs available may often dictate which statistical methods are used. The best general advice we can offer is that the statistical treatment given to data should be adequate and appropriate to address whatever hypotheses the experiments were designed to test.

The use of ISH in experiments where comparisons are made between data from animals in a number of treatment groups (including control or sham-treated groups) is a common application of this technique, and some guidelines for the analysis of these experiments are presented here. Firstly, films or emulsions should be sampled by an observer 'blind' to the treatment groups to prevent operator bias from influencing image analysis. Randomized coding of animals across groups, with the code only being revealed after sampling, is a simple way to achieve this objective. After image analysis, data (means ± S.E.M. for the parameters being studied) from each sampling region from all animals in a particular treatment group may be pooled to give group statistics (mean ± S.E.M.). Group data may then be compared in many ways. If a number of groups are being compared with a control group and/or with each other, multiple comparison procedures, which minimize the risk of making false inferences from multiple comparisons, should be employed (see Ludbrook (1991) for review and examples). As the variation between samples of biological material is often greater than that predicted by the normal distribution, non-parametric statistical procedures may be appropriate in many situations (Siegel, 1956).

7.7.2 Reporting of ISH methods and results

There is no standard method for the reporting of ISH experiments, and dramatic variations in the amount of information presented may be seen in the literature. As readers of reports dealing with ISH should be able to replicate the findings presented, more rather than less detail in the description of methods would be an advantage. To this end, researchers should accurately describe, or refer to accurate descriptions of, all the experimental and analytical methods employed. This attention to detail should also apply to the control procedures used; if the researcher has gone to the trouble of ensuring the specificity of the results presented, these details should not be omitted. Since, as we have previously explained, so many options are available for image analysis and statistical analysis of results, the procedures adopted for these important tasks also need to be detailed.

In reporting the results of ISH experiments, an accurate description of the findings seen, along with appropriate examples of the raw data obtained (i.e. photographs of film or emulsion images), are invaluable in conveying these results to the reader. Explanations (including statistics) of any experimental changes seen should also be accompanied by photographs illustrating these effects as well as appropriate graphs or tables.

7.7.3 Relative versus absolute measurements of mRNA abundance

The methods described in this article for the analysis of ISH are essentially only useful for the relative quantification of regional or cellular mRNA. It is possible, if the specific radioactivity of the probe and the efficiency of autoradiography are known, to calculate the number of hybrids/cell from film OD or emulsion grain density (see Lewis *et al.*, 1989). Relating this value to the absolute mRNA concentration is, however, extremely difficult and relies on a number of assumptions which may not be valid. In the case of ISH, the loss of mRNA during preparation of samples, the efficiency of hybridization and the fact that transected cells or neurons are used in hybridization are all factors that must cast doubt on the value of any absolute measurements. In addition, the response of X-ray film or nuclear emulsion to radioactivity is often unpredictable because of chemography, latent image fading and, if tritium is used, differential quenching (Rogers, 1979), further impeding attempts to obtain absolute measurements. In contrast, the relative quantification of ISH, using methods such as those presented here, has been extensively used by many research groups, and has provided meaningful results allowing comparison of many different tissues, developmental stages and experimental treatments.

7.8 RECENT DEVELOPMENTS AND FUTURE DIRECTIONS IN ISH

A number of new procedures and instruments have recently been implemented in ISH to increase the speed and/or resolution of this technique. Systems utilizing *storage phosphors* are now marketed by a number of manufacturers (e.g. Molecular Dynamics, Fuji, Kodak). Storage phosphor materials record the number of trapped electrons proportional to the radiation dose, and a characteristic visible light emission is produced when these electrons are released (upon stimulation with light or heat). In ISH, sections hybridized with radiolabelled probe (using any of the isotopes commonly employed) are apposed to imaging screens containing storage phosphor material. After this exposure (usually minutes to hours), the spatial pattern of electron release is recorded by an image reader (using a laser beam scanning system and photomultiplier tube) and analysed in the same way as X-ray film images. Compared with X-ray film methods, storage phosphors have the advantages of being faster, having a linear response to radioactivity over a wider range of values, and, in most cases, being reusable (Kuhar *et al.*, 1991). The need for the darkroom facilities and chemicals used with X-ray film techniques is also avoided by the use of storage phosphor imaging plates. The initial cost of these systems is currently relatively high, although the falling cost and the increasing range of options available suggests that they may well be widely used in the near future.

An autoradiography system recently introduced by Packard (the InstantImager) utilizes a *microchannel array detector* (MICAD) and *multiwire proportional counting* (MWPC) to record radioactive emissions from many isotopes (not tritium at present), providing quantitative spatial data at the regional level. Electrons emitted by radioactive specimens are sensed by an array of charged wire screens and then displayed as a spatial image of radioactive abundance. This technology reputedly provides even faster results than storage phosphor imaging plates (typically seconds to minutes) and also has a wider dynamic range. As is the case with systems utilizing storage phosphors, this equipment is becoming more affordable and more widely used.

Techniques involving *chemiluminescence* (e.g. Amersham's ECL system) are currently used for the analysis of DNA blots, and may soon be developed for use with ISH. These non-isotopic procedures utilize direct labelling of DNA probes with the enzyme horseradish peroxidase, and may in future provide cellular resolution with greater speed and sensitivity than current radioactive and non-isotopic ISH methods.

Advances in computer technology may soon see the arrival of more sophisticated image analysis hardware and software. Three-dimensional visualization of image data is now possible (though at a high price) through more powerful graphics and imaging processors. Programs such as Brain Browser (Academic Press, San Diego, U.S.A.), providing a computerized atlas of the rat brain and a database of neuronal circuitry, may be incorporated into IASs to provide faster and more reproducible sampling and analysis, and allowing three-dimensional maps of mRNA distribution to be built up.

7.9 CONCLUSION

The technique of ISH is a powerful tool in the study of factors regulating gene expression, and is in widespread use in the biological sciences and particularly in the field of neuroscience. The desire to measure the extent of apparent differences between experimental samples has led to the development of sophisticated computer analysis procedures, some of which have been discussed in the present work. Alterations in gene expression (as reflected by mRNA levels) involving an approximate halving or doubling (or more) of control mRNA levels have regularly been reported by many research groups in a variety of experimental models. Moreover, despite the inherent variability of the experimental techniques used in ISH, changes as small as 30% have been observed using properly applied ISH and computerized image analysis. With advances in ISH and computerized image analysis technology, the reproducibility and sensitivity of these techniques will no doubt improve even further.

ACKNOWLEDGEMENTS

Research in the authors' laboratory is supported by grants from the National Health and Medical Research Council (NH&MRC) of Australia and the William Buckland and Ian Potter Foundations. R.D.O. is the recipient of an NH&MRC Biomedical Postgraduate Research Scholarship.

REFERENCES

Armitage, P. & Berry, G. (1987) *Statistical Methods in Medical Research*, 2nd edn. Blackwell Scientific Publications, Oxford.

Augood, S.J., Faull, R.L. & Emson, P.C. (1992) *Eur. J. Neurosci.* **4**, 102–112.

Burton, K.A., Kabigting, E.B., Clifton, D.K. & Steiner, R.A. (1992) *Endocrinology* **130**, 958–963.

Dagerlind, Å., Friberg, K., Bean, A.J. & Hökfelt, T. (1992) *Histochemistry* **98**, 39–49.

Davenport, A.P. & Hall, M.D. (1988) *J. Neurosci. Methods* **25**, 75–82.

Davenport, A.P. & Nunez, D.J. (1990) In *In situ hybridization: principles and practice*. J.M. Polak & J. O'D. McGee (eds). Oxford University Press, Oxford. pp. 95–111.

Eilbert, J.L., Gallistel, C.R. & McEachron, D.L. (1990). *Comp. Med. Imag. Graph.* **14**, 331–339.

Emson, P.C. (1993). *Trends Neurosci.* **16**, 9–16.

Harlan, R.E., Shivers, B.D., Romano, G.J., Howells, R.D. & Pfaff, D.W. (1987). *J. Comp. Neurol.* **258**, 159–184.

Jablonski, E., Moomaw, E.W., Tullis, R.H. & Ruth, J. (1986). *Nucleic Acids Res.* **14**, 6115–6128.

Kuhar, M.J., De Souza, E.B. & Unnerstall, J.R. (1986). *Annu. Rev. Neurosci.* **9**, 27–59.

Kuhar, M.J., Lloyd, D.G., Appel, N. & Loats, H.L. (1991). *J. Chem. Neuroanat.* **4**, 319–327.

Lewis, M.E., Rogers, W.T., Krause II, R.G. & Schwaber, J.S. (1989). *Methods Enzymol.* **168**, 808–821.

Ludbrook, J. (1991). *Clin. Exp. Pharmacol. Physiol.* **18**, 379–392.

McCabe, J.T., Kao, T.-C. & Volkov, M.L. (1993). *Microsc. Res. Tech.* **25**, 61–67.

Paxinos, G. and Watson, C. (1986). *The rat brain in stereotaxic coordinates*, 2nd edn. Academic Press, Sydney.

Ramm, P. (1990) *Comp. Med. Imag. Graph.* **14**, 287–306.

Rogers, A.W. (1979). *Techniques of autoradiography*, 3rd edn. Elsevier, New York.

Rogers, W.T., Schwaber, J.S. & Lewis, M.E. (1987). *Neurosci. Lett.* **82**, 315–320.

Siegel, S. (1956). *Non-parametric statistics*. McGraw-Hill, New York.

Smolen, A.J. & Beaston-Wimmer, P. (1990). In '*In situ hybridization histochemistry*' (ed. M.-F. Chesselet), pp. 175–188. CRC Press, Boca Raton.

Sokal, R.R. & Rohlf, F.J. (1981). *Biometry*, 2nd edn. W.H. Freeman, New York.

Trembleau, A., Roche, D. & Calas, A. (1993). *J. Histochem. Cytochem.* **41**, 489–498.

Uhl, G.R. (1989). *Methods Enzymol.* **168**, 741–752.

Uhl, G.R. & Nishimori, T. (1990). *Cell. Mol. Neurobiol.* **10**, 73–98.

Weiss, L.T. & Chesselet, M.-F. (1989). *Mol. Brain Res.* **5**, 121–130.

Young, W.S. III. (1990). In *Handbook of chemical neuroanatomy*, Vol. 8: *Analysis of neuronal microcircuits and synaptic interactions*' (eds. A. Björklund, T. Hökfelt, F.G. Wouterlood & A.N. van den Pol), pp. 481–512. Elsevier, Amsterdam.

PART II

Non-radioactive *in situ* Hybridization Methods

Non-radioactive *in situ* hybridization using alkaline phosphatase-labelled oligonucleotides

S.J. AUGOOD*, E.M. McGOWAN*, B.R FINSEN†,
B. HEPPELMAN‡ & P.C. EMSON*

* MRC Molecular Neuroscience Group, Department of Neurobiology, AFRC Babraham Institute,
Cambridge CB2 4AT, UK
† PharmaBiotec Research Center, Institute of Neurobiology, University of Aarhus, DK-8000 Aarhus
C, Denmark
‡ Physiologisches Institut, Universität Würzburg, Röntgenring 9, D-8700, Würzburg, Germany

8.1 INTRODUCTION TO ALKALINE PHOSPHATASE-LABELLED OLIGONUCLEOTIDES

In the search to make classical radioactive *in situ* hybridization (ISH) methods using 3′-tailed synthetic oligonucleotides less complex and more accessible to researchers without radiochemical facilities, various non-radioactive methods have been developed. In most cases, the synthetic oligonucleotide is tagged with a reporter molecule, such as biotin or mercury, at the 3′ or 5′ end (Langer *et al.*, 1981; Agrawal *et al.*, 1986; Hopman *et al.*, 1986), and then the sites of hybridization are visualized using a suitable detection system, for example, a streptavidin antibody complex. Although many of these 'indirect' *in situ* methods are sensitive and give excellent results on membrane blots and tissue sections, they may be more suited to qualitative rather than quantitative studies, as the detection procedure involves several amplification steps.

In our experience, for both qualitative and semiquantitative studies, alkaline phosphatase (AP)-labelled oligonucleotides are the probes of choice for non-radioactive studies. Although these probes offer many advantages over their non-radioactive adversaries, and indeed radio-labelled oligonucleotides, they do have their limitations. In our hands, AP probes (i) give excellent cellular resolution of hybridization sites on tissue sections (Kiyama & Emson, 1990; Kiyama *et al.*, 1990a; Augood *et al.*, 1991a,b, 1992; Augood & Emson, 1992) and neuronal cultures (Finsen *et al.*, 1992) (a particulate signal is detected in the cell cytoplasm, the definition of the signal being dependent upon the thickness of the tissue section, the thinner the section the more cellular detail is visible), (ii) may be purchased commercially and stored at 4°C for at least 12 months without loss of enzyme activity, (iii) are easy to use (no additional detection kit/antibody complex is required to detect sites of probe hybridization), (iv) are fast (the AP hybridization signal is detected within 12–48 h

IN SITU HYBRIDIZATION PROTOCOLS FOR THE BRAIN
ISBN 0–12–759919–3

after washing of the sections), (v) may be used for semiquantitative analysis as no amplification steps are involved; the intensity of the AP hybridization signal is directly proportional to the amount of probe hybridized (therefore the amount of mRNA present)), (vi) may be combined with radioactive oligonucleotides (^{35}S and possibly ^{33}P) and antibodies for co-expression and co-localization studies, and (vii), in our hands at least, are more sensitive than other non-radioactive counterparts. The disadvantages are less numerous, yet just as important: (i) these oligonucleotides are not as sensitive as ^{35}S-labelled oligonucleotides when detecting rare transcripts, (ii) they will not work to give the optimal hybridization signal without modification of the standard hybridization conditions given in Chapter 1, (iii) they are still relatively expensive to purchase (the purity of the labelled probe varies considerably and is dependent on the supplier) and (iv) although several 'user-friendly' labelling kits are available, in our experience, the end product often requires further purification, e.g. fast protein liquid chromatography (FPLC). For a list of kit suppliers, the reader should refer to Emson (1993).

8.1.1 Synthesis and labelling of AP-oligonucleotides

In 1986 Jablonski and colleagues reported a method for covalently cross-linking calf intestinal AP to short (21–26 mers) synthetic oligonucleotides. This was one of the first 'direct' non-radioactive methods to be reported. A simplified overview of their method of labelling with AP is given below; some modifications have been incorporated. A modified thymine base terminating in a reactive primary amine is incorporated directly into the automated oligonucleotide synthesis; the modified oligonucleotide is then reacted with the homobifunctional reagent, disuccinimidyl suberate (pH > 7), and the reaction allowed to proceed for 5 min in the dark: the reaction mixture is then applied to a Sephadex G-25 column, eluted with water, immediately frozen and lyophilized. The activated linker arm oligonucleotide is then rehydrated with a 2-fold excess of AP and the conjugation

reaction is left to proceed for 16 h at room temperature. Finally protein products are separated from non-protein components by gel filtration, while the pure AP-oligonucleotide conjugate is separated from free AP by FPLC. The purified end product is then concentrated using a Minicon Macrosolute Concentrator (Amicon). This chemical procedure is discussed in detail elsewhere (Kadowaki *et al.*, 1993).

8.1.2 Storage of AP-oligonucleotides

AP-oligonucleotides should not be frozen and should be stored at 4°C, as recommended by the manufacturers. To preserve the activity of the enzyme, we store our AP-oligonucleotides in buffer containing 30 mM Tris, 3.0 M NaCl, 1.0 mM $MgCl_2$, 0.1 mM $ZnCl_2$ and 0.05% sodium azide, pH 7.6 at 4°C. Once these oligonucleotides have been diluted in hybridization buffer, they should be used immediately. They should *never* be stored for long periods in the presence of formamide, for example diluted in hybridization buffer, because formamide (> 36 h) significantly reduces the activity of the enzyme and therefore reduces the intensity of the final hybridization signal.

8.2 PREPARATION OF FRESH FROZEN CNS TISSUE SECTIONS

Once the brain has been removed from the skull, and frozen as described in Chapter 1 (Section 1.2), we have found it best to thaw–mount cryostat sections (10–15 μm) on to gelatin–chrom alum-coated slides. Alternative adhesion substrates may be used, such as poly(L-lysine) or Vectabond (Vector Labs); however, silating agents tend to inhibit AP enzyme activity and can result in a reduced AP hybridization signal. The recipe for preparing gelatin-coated slides is given in Protocol 8.1.

8.2.1 Preparation of paraffin-embedded CNS tissue sections

For qualitative studies of gene expression, paraffin-embedded semi-thin (5–7 μm) sections

Protocol 8.1 Preparation of gelatin–chrom alum-coated slides.

1. Wearing gloves, load microscope slides[a] into glass staining racks[b].
2. Rinse slides in acetone (5 min) and air-dry.
3. Warm 500 ml of DEPC-treated water to 50°C then add 5 g of gelatin powder and 0.25 g of chromic potassium sulphate. Stir until dissolved.
4. Filter solution and allow to cool to 37°C; dip slides in glass slide racks into the warm gelatin solution for 3 min, remove and drain off excess.
5. Leave slides to dry in an oven for several hours.
6. Coated slides may be stored for several weeks in partitioned slide boxes.

[a] For convenience we use twin-frosted precleaned slides from Solmedia.
[b] It is advisable to keep a set of glass slide racks which are used exclusively for coating as the gelatin hardens on to the racks and a substantial deposit can build up. Gelatin–chrom alum solution may be reused. Filter the solution, autoclave and store at 4°C. Before subbing the slides, warm the gelatin solution to 37–42°C (we routinely do this in a microwave).

Protocol 8.2 Paraffin embedding of tissue blocks (routine processing by machine).

1. Fix tissue in 4% paraformaldehyde for up to 24 h (largely dependent on size of tissue).
2. Dehydrate through ethanol: 50% (12 h), 70% (12 h), 90% (3 h), 2 × 100% (1.5 h each), fresh 100% (2 h), then delipidate in chloroform: I, 3 h; II, 8 h[a].
3. Impregnate tissue with paraffin wax (60°C): use three changes of wax, 1 h each (last change in a vacuum bath) before finally embedding in fresh wax (60°C) in a cast.
4. Allow wax to set, remove wax block from plastic moulding and trim excess paraffin. Before cutting, allow block to stand on ice (cut face down).
5. Cut ribbons of 5–7 μm sections, float out on to the surface of a warm water bath (to allow sections to unravel), when sections completely flat, mount on to coated slides[b] and dry. Sections may then be stored at room temperature for several months.

Rapid processing for small tissue (e.g. dorsal root ganglia)

1. Fix tissue in 4% paraformaldehyde[c] and dehydrate: 50% (1 h), 70% (1 h), 90% (1 h), 100% twice 45 min each.
2. Delipidate tissue with benzene/toluene twice 15–45 min per change.
3. Impregnate with warm paraffin wax 2 × 1 h, then embed in fresh wax as above.

[a] Tissue may stay in chloroform for longer than 8 h.
[b] Gelatin–chrom alum-coated slides are not recommended here as the sections are already fixed, so tissue proteins will not cross-link with the gelatin and hold the sections in place; consequently sections will float off. Alternative substrates that may be used for paraffin sections include Vectabond (Vector Labs) or 3-aminopropyltriethoxysilane (APES; Sigma; A-3648).
[c] If tissue is fixed in Bouin's fluid, then miss out 50% ethanol and go straight to 70% ethanol.

offer excellent cellular resolution of the AP-hybridization signal combined with preserved tissue morphology (see Figure 8.1). Furthermore, after development of the coloured AP reaction product, sections may be processed for immunocytochemistry allowing antigens and mRNA to be simultaneously visualized in the same tissue section (see Section 8.8; Emson *et al.*, 1993; Heppelman *et al.*, 1993). In our experience it is preferable to carry out the ISH first and the immunocytochemistry subsequently; however, this ordering depends on the stability of the antigen; for the localization of oestrogen receptor immunoreactivity in the cell nucleus, for example, it may be better to carry out the immunocytochemistry procedure first (using sterile conditions and diethyl pyrocarbonate

(DEPC)-treated buffers) and the AP ISH second (A. Herbison, personal communication). The ordering of the two steps should be determined for each antibody. We have had most success performing the immunocytochemistry second.

Paraffin-embedded blocks are prepared using a routine method. For CNS tissue, rodents are first anaesthetized with Sagattal, perfused transcardially with freshly prepared ice-cold heparinized (1%, v/v) DEPC-treated saline followed by 4% neutral buffered paraformaldehyde in 0.1 M phosphate-buffered saline (PBS); tissue blocks are then postfixed overnight. Submersion of fixed tissue may also be used, for example, post-mortem human blocks, but the morphology is, as expected, not as well preserved. Blocks are then processed as standard (see Protocol 8.2).

There are several advantages to be gained from using paraffin-embedded tissue for ISH studies: (i) the morphology of the sections is excellent and allows clear observation of the cellular localization of the AP hybridization signal, usually seen as a particulate 'hot spot' within the cell cytoplasm of thin (5–7 μm) sections; (ii) it allows access to a vast archive of human post-mortem tissue collected and processed for routine histological studies; and (iii) tissue sections may be cut, mounted on to RNAse-free coated slides and stored at room temperature for several months (if not longer) without any deterioration in hybridization signal.

8.2.2 Preparation of neuronal cultures

When applying AP ISH to neuronal cultures (see Figure 8.2 for example), it is important to ensure that (i) the cultures are grown on a support medium which may be used directly in the hybridization process, (ii) that this support medium is pretreated with a substrate that will ensure that the cultures will not float off during the relatively high-temperature (55°C) post-hybridization washes, and (iii) that this substrate is relatively inert and will not adversely affect the developing cultures. To this end we grow both dispersed primary cultures and CNS slice explants on poly(L-lysine)-coated glass coverslips (Chapter 1; Protocol 1.1). Routinely, explants are from P0–P7 Wistar rat pups; tissue slices are

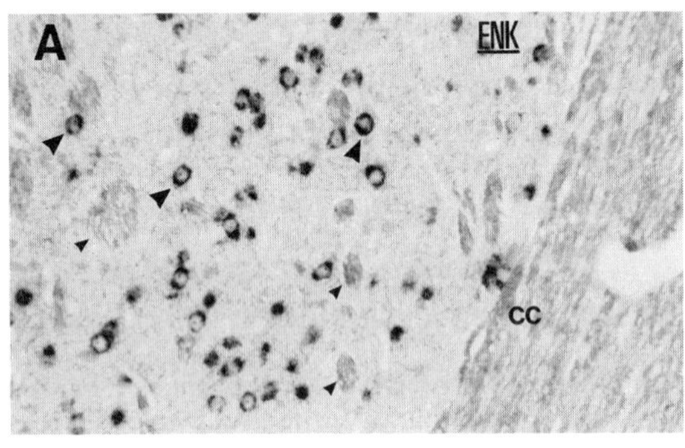

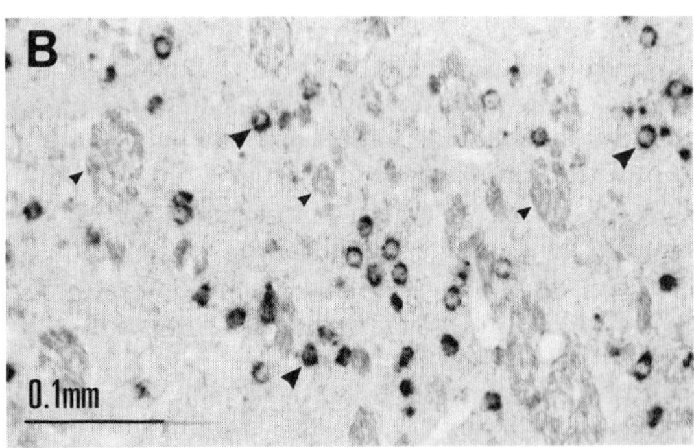

Figure 8.1 Semi-thin (7 μm) sections of paraffin-embedded rat striatum hybridized with AP-labelled oligonucleotide complementary to a portion of the rat pre-proenkephalin A (ENK) mRNA. The AP-reaction product is concentrated in the cell cytoplasm whereas the cell nuclei are relatively devoid of signal, illustrated by large arrowheads in both (A) and (B); the smaller arrowheads indicate fibre bundles in the striatum. cc, corpus callosum.

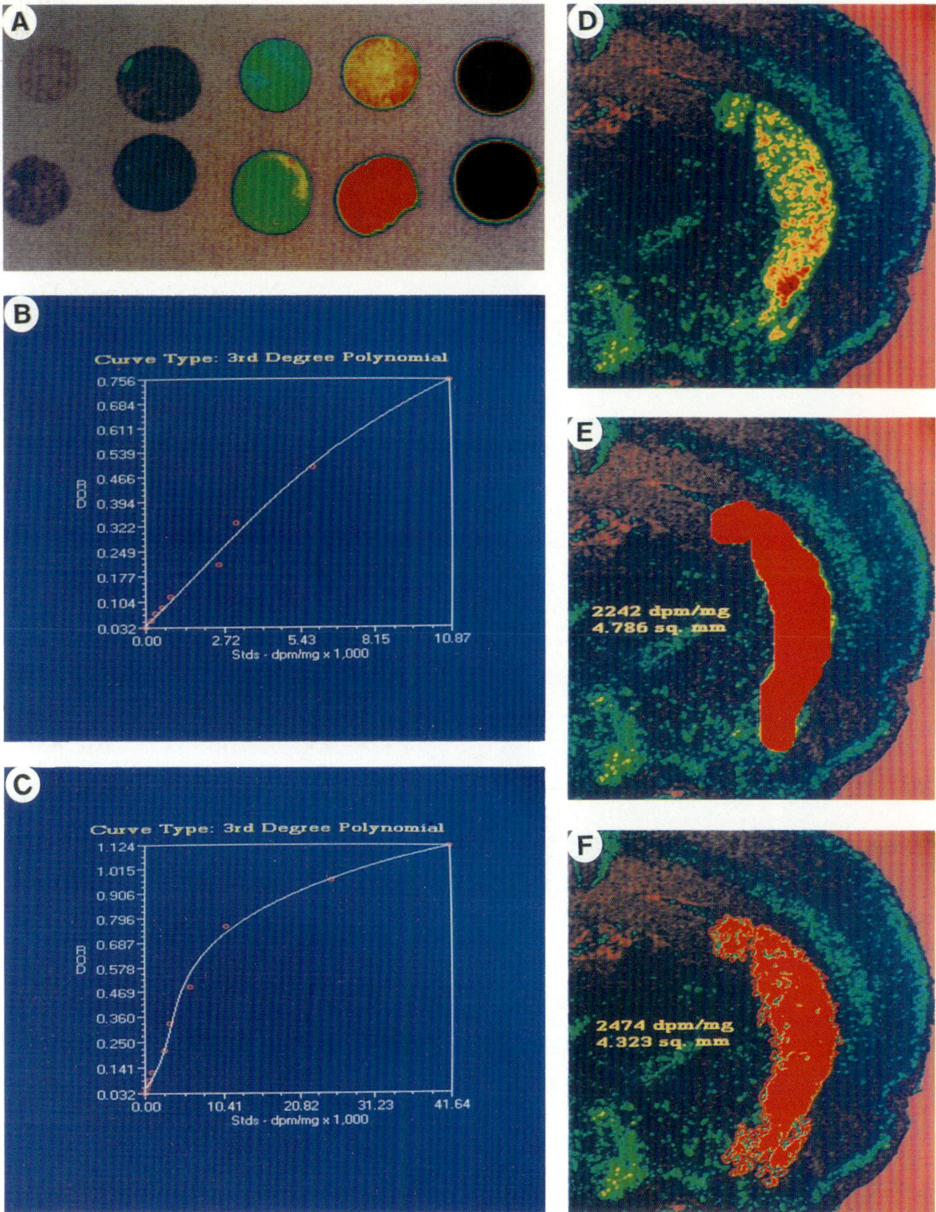

Colour Plate 1 (A) Pseudocolour representation of an X-ray film image of ^{35}S-labelled brain paste standards prepared using the method of Protocol 7.1. Density values range from pink (170 d.p.m. mg^{-1}), through blue, green, yellow and red to black (42 000 d.p.m. mg^{-1}). (B) Calibration curve constructed from standards 1–8 from (A). Note that the curve is essentially linear over the OD range 0.05–0.75. Third-degree polynomial was chosen as the best fit in this case. (C) Calibration curve constructed from all ten standards from (A). The curve is non-linear above OD 0.8 when darkest standards are included. The range of linear values varies for different film types, IASs and calibration conditions. (D) Pseudocolour representation of X-ray film image of pre-proenkephalin mRNA localization in 14 μm section of rat forebrain. Pink represents lowest OD values (background in this case), while red is highest. (E) Manual outlining of striatum from (D), with corresponding density and area measurements superimposed. (F) Automatic sampling of striatum from (D). Note higher average density and lower area values compared with those from manual outlining, because of patches of tissue below threshold value being omitted from sampling. Area × density values from manual and automatic sampling are virtually identical in this case.

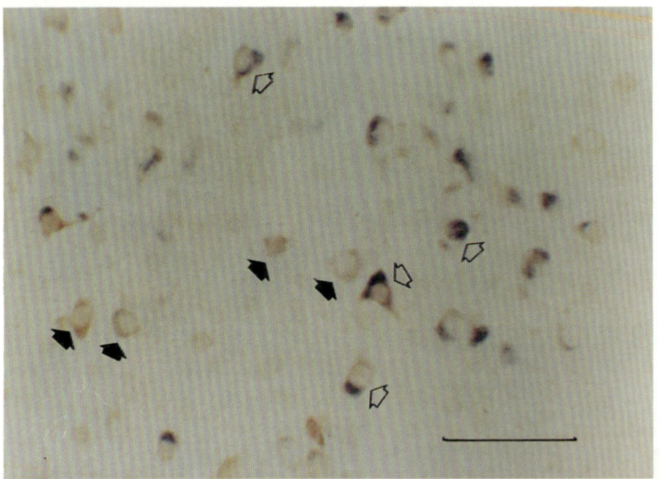

Colour Plate 2 Colour Photomicrograph demonstrating the co-localization of calretinin mRNA (purple reaction product) and calbindin-D28K immunoreactivity (brown diaminobenzidine product) in a paraffin-embedded section of rat substantia nigra. Most neurons in the substantia nigra contain calbindin-D28K (closed arrows) and a subpopulation of these neurons also express calretinin mRNA (open arrows). Scale bar = 75 μm.

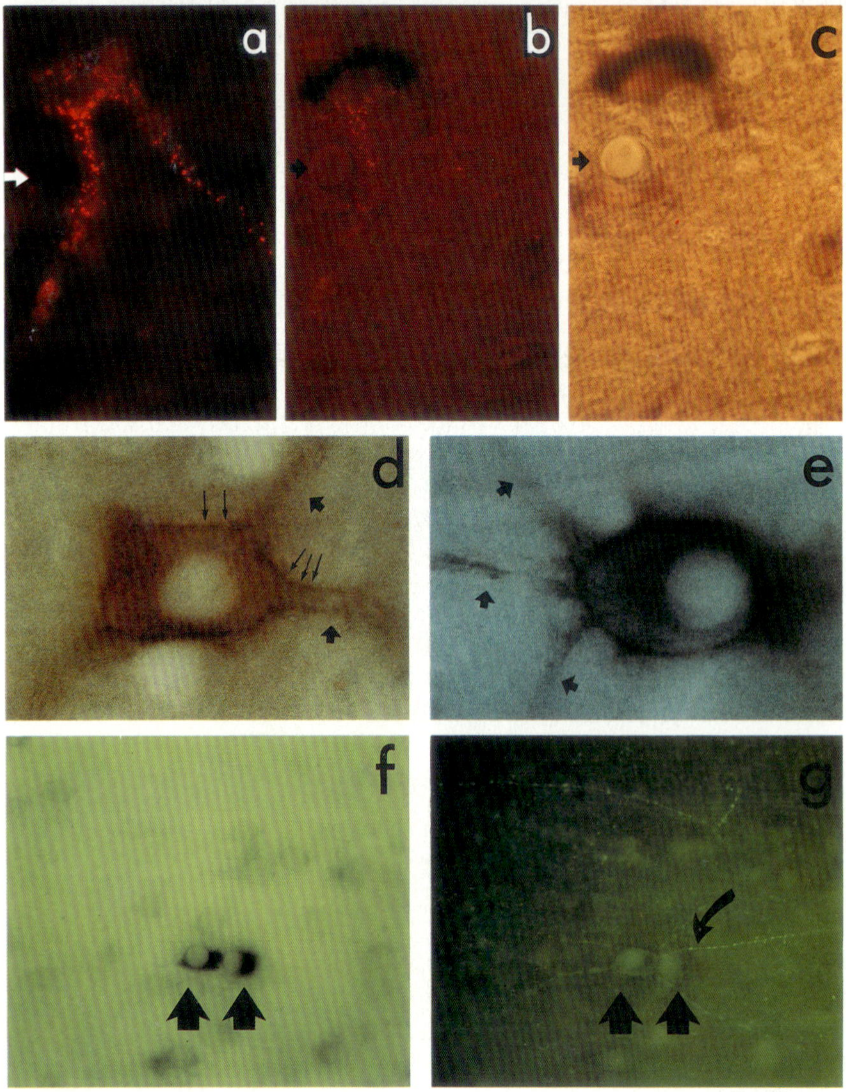

Colour Plate 3 Double-labelling experiments. (a) Retrogradely transported rhodamin-conjugated latex beads visualized with fluorescence have accumulated in the soma and dendrites of a neuron in the cat's nucleus of the optic tract. (b) GAD mRNA was visualized, and both products can be seen in a mixed exposure. (c) Brightfield exposure shows the AP reaction product in this neuron. (d) GAD mRNA, red reaction product, in a VVA lectin-labelled neuron. (e) Same as in (d) but blue reaction product. Neurons were from adult cat visual cortex. Fat arrows point to labelled processes, the fine arrows indicate the typical fenestrated VVA-labelling pattern. (f, g) Organotypic culture (explanted at postnatal day 2 and maintained for 2 weeks *in vitro*) of rat visual cortex displays NPY mRNA-expressing neurons (f, the bold arrows) which co-localize NPY-immunoreactive material, as revealed with FITC-labelled secondary antibody (g). The curved arrow points to the axon of one cell. Note the many immunoreactive beaded processes and puncta indicating the dense NPY innervation of the culture.

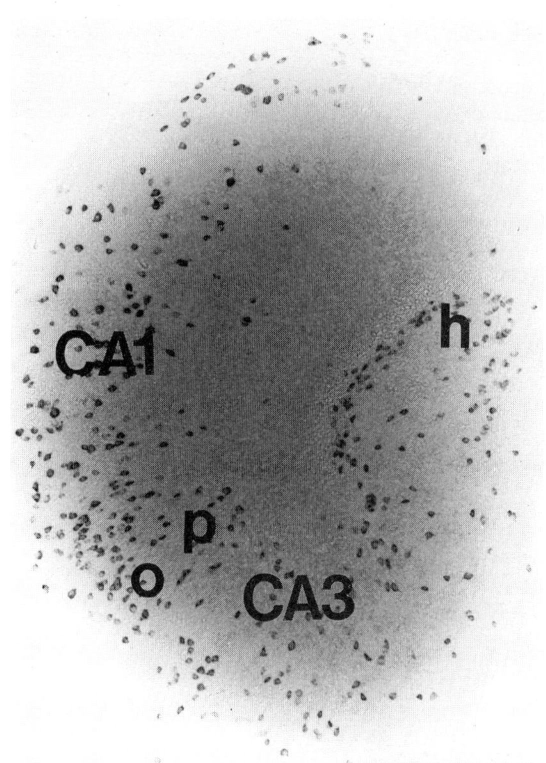

Figure 8.2 Somatostatin (SRIF) gene expression in 5-week-old whole hippocampal explant culture. Note the high numbers of organotypically distributed neurons throughout the hippocampal fields. The number and distribution of neurons detected by the AP-SRIF probe is, in essence, identical with that revealed by immunocytochemistry using an anti-SRIF antibody (Finsen *et al.*, 1992). h, dentate hilus; o, stratum oriens; p, stratum pyramidale. Scale bar = 400 μm.

cut (350 μm) using a McIlwain tissue chopper and then placed individually on coverslips in a drop of chicken plasma, coagulated by thrombin and then grown for 4–5 weeks using the roller tube technique (Gähwiler, 1981, 1984). Detailed protocols describing the culturing of CNS explants are provided elsewhere (Østergaard *et al.*, 1990, 1991). Immediately before processing, coverslips are removed from the roller tube and either fixed as complete cultures or snap-frozen on dry ice and sectioned on a cryostat (14 μm), thaw-mounted on to gelatin-coated coverslips and processed for ISH as standard (Finsen *et al.*, 1992).

8.3 HYBRIDIZATION

We have found that the activity of these enzyme-conjugated oligonucleotides may be significantly affected by a multitude of variables, the quality of deionized distilled water being critical for optimal results. To avoid unnecessary 'variables' we always use deionized double-distilled Milli Q water for all stages of hybridization. Contamination of the water or buffers by heavy metal ions or related 'gremlins' can significantly affect the strength of the resulting AP hybridization signal, to the point when no signal at all will be detected! All Milli-Q water is treated with the RNAse inhibitor, diethylpyrocarbonate (DEPC), as described in Chapter 1, and autoclaved before use. We tend to err on the side of caution and treat most buffers with DEPC; as mentioned earlier in Chapter 1, such cautionary steps may not be necessary but old habits die hard!

8.3.1 Estimating optimal hybridization and washing conditions

For oligonucleotides, optimal conditions, for example hybridization and washing temperatures, may be calculated empirically and are dependent upon the length of the probe, the GC content, the Na^+ concentration and the percentage of deionized formamide used. To determine the optimal conditions, it is important to determine the temperature at which 50% of DNA–RNA duplexes dissociate (referred to as the T_m). An estimation of the T_m for each oligonucleotide can be determined using the following basic equation (Wilkinson, 1992):

$$T_m \; (°C) = 79.8 + 18.5 \log(\text{molarity of monovalent cations}) + 0.58(\% \; G+C) + 0.12(\% \; G+C)^2 - 0.5(\% \; \text{formamide}) - (820 \div \text{probe length in bp})$$

This equation should be used as a guide only, as it applies to DNA–RNA hybrids formed in solution and it is important to realize that the hybrids formed during ISH on fixed tissue are less stable and will therefore have an actual melting temperature slightly lower than the theoretical value calculated using the above formula.

Protocol 8.3 Standard hybridization protocol for fresh
frozen sections.

1. Remove sections from −80°C freezer and dry with a hair dryer.
2. Fix, dehydrate and air-dry as in Chapter 1.
3. Remove hybridization buffer from −20°C freezer and keep on ice.
   Hybridization buffer[a] contains: 50% deionized formamide[b], 10%
   dextran sulphate, 4×SSC, 1×Denhardt's soln[c] and 250 μg ml^{-1}
   sonicated salmon testis DNA[d] (Dithiothreitol is not necessary as no ^{35}S
   is present; it also inhibits AP activity).
4. Dilute AP-oligonucleotide in hybridization buffer. *Do not boil the
   probe*. Vortex *well*, return to ice and allow bubbles to clear before
   pipetting 250 μl of diluted probe on to each slide. Spread the buffer
   carefully over the sections using an 'upturned' yellow Gilson pipette
   tip being careful not to scratch the tissue.
5. Place plastic trays in humidified plastic bags and hybridize overnight
   (12–36 h, but no longer) at 37°C.

[a] This is a compromise between the 'minimalist' and 'maximalist' hybridization
buffers described in Chapter 1; large volumes (40 ml) can be made up and stored
at −20°C.
[b] It is imperative to maintain the activity of the AP at all times so it is recommended
that the formamide be deionized using Amberlite M-80 resin (Sigma). Radioactive
oligonucleotides are less sensitive to stray contaminations, such as metal ions,
than AP-probes. Mix 100 ml of formamide with 5 g of resin and stir gently at
room temperature for 1 h in a sterile beaker. Filter the deionized formamide
twice and store in 20 ml aliquots at −20°C.
[c] For convenience use RNAse-free Denhardt's solution (Sigma D-2532) and
[d] RNAse-free DNA (Sigma D-9156) and store frozen.

The optimal incubation temperature for anneal-
ing is 10–15°C below the T_m for 50% formamide;
for AP-oligonucleotides the true value of T_m is
approximately 10°C lower than the empirical
value.

8.3.2 Hybridization to fresh frozen sections

In this section, variations on the standard
radioactive ISH protocol (Chapter 1; Protocols
1.5 and 1.6) will be described and explanations
offered for the modifications. The method that
we have found to work well for most AP-
oligonucleotides is given in Protocol 8.3. In brief,
fresh frozen sections are taken from the −80°C
freezer just before the experiment, warmed to
room temperature, then fixed and dehydrated as
described in Chapter 1, air-dried and overlaid
with hybridization buffer containing the diluted
AP-oligonucleotide. It is important to dilute the
AP-oligonucleotide in hybridization buffer just
before application (see Section 8.2). Routinely
we cover sections with 250 μl of buffer per slide
(containing three to four sections). AP-oligonucleotides are diluted to give a final saturating
probe concentration of 6–12 fmol μl^{-1} (1–2 μl ml^{-1}
of 2 nmol in 200 μl of stock). This probe
concentration is saturating for most neuropeptide, transmitter and receptor transcripts in CNS
tissue but may need to be increased for detection
of very abundant transcripts, for example actin
mRNA. It is important to use saturating probe
concentrations to ensure that there is sufficient
probe to bind to all available hybridization sites;
this criterion *must* be satisified for semiquantitative analysis of ISH data (see Section 8.5).
Sections are hybridized overnight at 37°C in
humidified plastic/Perspex trays (Nunc cat. no.
166508). The trays are sealed inside a plastic bag
containing several 'water soggy' paper towels and
placed in an incubator/oven humidified by pots
of distilled water. It is important that the sections
do not dry out at all during this and any
subsequent steps as this will lead to an increase
in background staining and the 'dried out'

Protocol 8.4 Using paraffin-embedded sections.

1. Heat a hot-plate with a flat surface to > 60°C.
2. Take slide containing the mounted sections and quicky place on hot-plate (section side up) until the paraffin wax melts (wax surrounding the embedded tissue will become transparent). This should take approx. 90 s for a section of rat CNS tissue.
3. Quickly, before wax re-sets, dissolve wax in xylene (2 × 5 min).
4. Partially rehydrate sections, 100%, 90%, 70% ethanol (2 × 5 min each).
5. Rinse in 0.1 M PBS (10 min).
6. Overlay sections with 0.02% pepsin in 0.2 M HCl and incubate at 37°C for 30 min.
7. Refix sections with 4% paraformaldehyde in 0.1 M PBS (pH 7.4) for 30 min.
8. Rinse sections in 0.2% glycine in 0.1 M PBS (3 × 5 min).
9. Finally sections may be dehydrated, air-dried and overlaid with hybridization buffer as described in Protocol 8.3.

portion of the section/s turning purple/black during the subsequent colour-development stage.

8.3.3 Hybridization to paraffin-embedded sections

There are numerous methods (Hoefler *et al.*, 1986; Wolber and Lloyd, 1988; Brahic & Haase, 1989; Pringle *et al.*, 1989) for localizing mRNA within paraffin-embedded tissue; many are variations on a 'standard' protocol. Assuming that the tissue has been fixed, processed and sectioned to yield relatively intact mRNA, it is important to include in the protocol a proteinase step which allows the oligonucleotide access to the target transcript. The method that we have found to be successful for a variety of applications (for combining with antibody and radioactive ISH studies, for example) is given in Protocol 8.4.

8.4 POST-HYBRIDIZATION WASHING AND COLOUR DEVELOPMENT

For AP-labelled oligonucleotides (26–36 mers), we routinely wash hybridized sections according to a standard protocol: one-room temperature rinse in 1×SSC followed by three washes in 1×SSC at 55°C (30 min each). Higher-temperature washes, especially in the presence of lauryl sulphate (SDS), are not advisable as this can result in sections floating off the gelatinized slides as well as in inhibition of AP enzyme activity. As noted in Chapter 1 (Section 1.4.2), it is probably the stringency of the hybridization that is critical in determining the specificity of the final hybridization signal. If the washing temperature is increased too much, the T_m of the oligonucleotide will be reached and all the specific DNA–RNA hybrids will melt. It is important to remember that AP-labelled oligonucleotides have an actual T_m some 10°C below the empirical value (see Section 8.3.1). After the final 1×SSC 55°C wash, sections are rinsed in 1×SSC at room temperature, then rinsed in a Tris buffer before being overlaid with AP substrate solution and incubated overnight at 25°C in the dark. Again, in the UK especially during the winter months, it is important that this stage is carried out in a humidified incubator; room-temperature incubations are fine in warmer climates (21–26°C)!! A recipe detailing the washing conditions and subsequent colour development is given in Protocol 8.5.

The intensity of the hybridization signal can be monitored by viewing slides under the light microscope (do not let sections dry out). When neuropeptide mRNAs in CNS tissue are being visualized, colour-development times can vary from 4 to 36 h, depending on the abundance of the mRNA. Sections may be dehydrated rapidly using acetone; however, dehydrating with absolute

Protocol 8.5 Post-hybridization washing and colour development.

1. Remove hybridized sections from the incubator, collect an aliquot of the discarded hybridization buffer[a] and rinse sections briefly in $1 \times SSC$ at room temperature.
2. In a water bath at 55°C, wash sections three times with $1 \times SSC$ 30 min each wash.
3. Allow sections to cool in $1 \times SSC$ (approx. 30–60 min), then rinse in Buffer A[b] (pH 7.4) for 30 min, then freshly prepared Buffer B[c] (pH 9.4) for 5 min.
4. During the Buffer B rinse, prepare the AP substrate solution; for a standard 26 mm × 76 mm slide, 0.7 ml of substrate solution per slide is sufficient. From the number of slides calculate the total volume of substrate solution required, then immediately before use add 4.5 µl of NBT stock[d] and 3.5 µl of BCIP stock[e] per ml of Buffer B required.
5. Remove slides, one at a time, from the Buffer B wash, lay them horizontally in incubation trays and overlay them with 0.7 ml of substrate solution. Ensure the tray is kept level at all times during the colour-development stage. *Do not let the sections dry out during this stage* as this will result in non-specific staining.
6. Finally, place slides in the dark at 25°C and leave the colour reaction to proceed.
7. The colour reaction can be terminated by washing sections in Stop buffer[f].
8. Coverslip sections using glycerin jelly and store at 4°C to prevent gradual fading of the AP reaction product.

[a] Collect an aliquot of 'used' hybridization buffer containing the AP probe in an Eppendorf tube and during the colour development stage add approx. 0.5 ml of AP substrate solution to this solution. The solution in the Eppendorf tube should go dark blue within 1–2 h. This test tells you that the substrate solution is OK, the pH of Buffer B is OK, and that the AP probe was added in excess. If this test tube does not go blue overnight you are unlikely to see any specific AP hybridization signal on the tissue sections.
[b] Buffer A: 100 mM Tris/HCl + 150 mM NaCl: pH 7.4.
[c] Buffer B: 100 mM Tris/HCl + 100 mM NaCl + 50 mM $MgCl_2$: pH 9.4.
[d] To make up a stock NBT (nitroblue tetrazolium) solution dissolve 75 mg of NBT chloride (Boehringer-Mannheim 1087-479) in 1 ml of 70% dimethylformamide; prepare in a glass tube only. Store in the dark at −20°C.
[e] To make up a stock solution of BCIP (5-bromo-4-chloro-3-indolyl-phosphate) dissolve 50 mg of BCIP toluidine salt (Boehringer-Mannheim 760-994) in 1 ml of 100% dimethylformamide. Store as above.
[f] Stop buffer: 100 mM Tris/HCl + 20 mM EDTA(Na_2) + 150 mM NaCl: pH 7.0–7.4.

alcohol will significantly reduce the intensity of the AP hybridization signal as the reaction product is alcohol soluble.

8.4.1 Variables affecting the intensity of AP hybridization signal

8.4.1.1 Formamide

As mentioned earlier, formamide inhibits both calf intestinal (source of AP for the AP-oligonucleotides) and endogenous AP activity in rat. Determining the fine balance between a strong specific hybridization signal and a low background is important. Routinely, commercial producers of AP-oligonucleotides recommend that the hybridization buffer should contain only 20% formamide; however, such a low concentration can often result in high non-specific background staining. For membrane blots this may not be a problem but for ISH on tissue sections, high background staining can often 'mask' the specific signal. To obtain the best

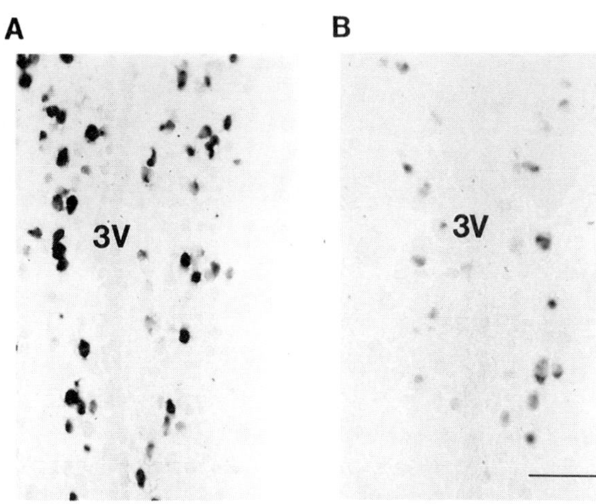

Figure 8.3 The effect of differing Mg^{2+} concentrations on the intensity of the AP signal. (A) Detection of SRIF mRNA in the periventricular region of the rat hypothalamus using a final concentration of 50 mM Mg^{2+} in the colour reaction buffer; (B) a serial section of hypothalamus hybridized and developed as in (A) but with only 5 mM Mg^{2+} in the final buffer. Both the number of cells detected and the intensity of the signal is much greater when using buffer containing 50 mM Mg^{2+}. 3V, third ventricle. Scale bar = 100 μm.

signal/noise ratio, we always test all AP-oligonucleotides using a range of formamide concentrations in the hybridization buffer; usually 30–50% formamide yields the best results using our standard protocol. Post-hybridization sections are never washed in the presence of formamide.

8.4.1.2 *pH of Buffer B and MgCl₂ concentration*

Both the pH and Mg^{2+} ion concentration of Buffer B are important. If the $[Mg^{2+}]$ is too low or the final pH of Buffer B is not in the range 9.0–9.5, then the rate at which the colour reaction proceeds will be hindered and the intensity of the coloured AP reaction product, depicting sites of hybridization, will be very weak or possibly undetectable. From various pilot experiments, we have determined that the optimal $[Mg^{2+}]$ is ~50 mM. Figure 8.3 illustrates this point.

8.4.1.3 *Number of oligonucleotides*

As with radioactive ISH, the intensity of the hybridization signal (and therefore the speed at which a signal is detected) may be markedly increased by hybridizing tissue sections with a mixture of several AP-oligonucleotides, each one being complementary to a different region of the transcript of interest. This approach is often adopted to visualize dopamine receptor mRNAs or other rare transcripts in brain using multiple radioactive oligonucleotides. Figure 8.4 demonstrates detection of calbindin mRNA in the rat cerebellum using either one or four AP-labelled oligonucleotides and compares this with four conventionally radiolabelled probes complementary to the same bases used in the design of the AP-labelled oligonucleotides.

8.5 USE OF AP-OLIGONUCLEOTIDES FOR SEMI-QUANTITATIVE ANALYSIS

If AP-oligonucleotides are to be used for semiquantitative analysis, for example, as tools for assessing relative changes in the cellular content of an mRNA after pharmacological manipulation, it is important to (i) ensure that saturating probe concentrations are used, (ii) process all control and experimental sections together to ensure that all hybridization and colour-development conditions are standardized, and (iii) establish a colour-development time course profile for each AP-oligonucleotide in the anatomical region of interest. An example of a colour-development time course profile is illustrated in Figure 8.5 showing that the intensity of the coloured AP hybridization signal increases linearly with time until 48 h, when the signal begins to plateau. Once the maximal intensity of signal is reached, the effective signal/noise ratio decreases as the intensity of the specific AP signal remains the same, whilst the level of background tissue staining increases with time. Colour-development times should not be extended beyond this point.

We have used AP-oligonucleotides for semi-quantitative analysis to assess the relative changes in cellular neuropeptide/transmitter mRNA content after several pharmacological manipulations (Kiyama *et al.*, 1990b; Augood *et al.*, 1991a,b, 1992; Augood & Emson, 1992). As

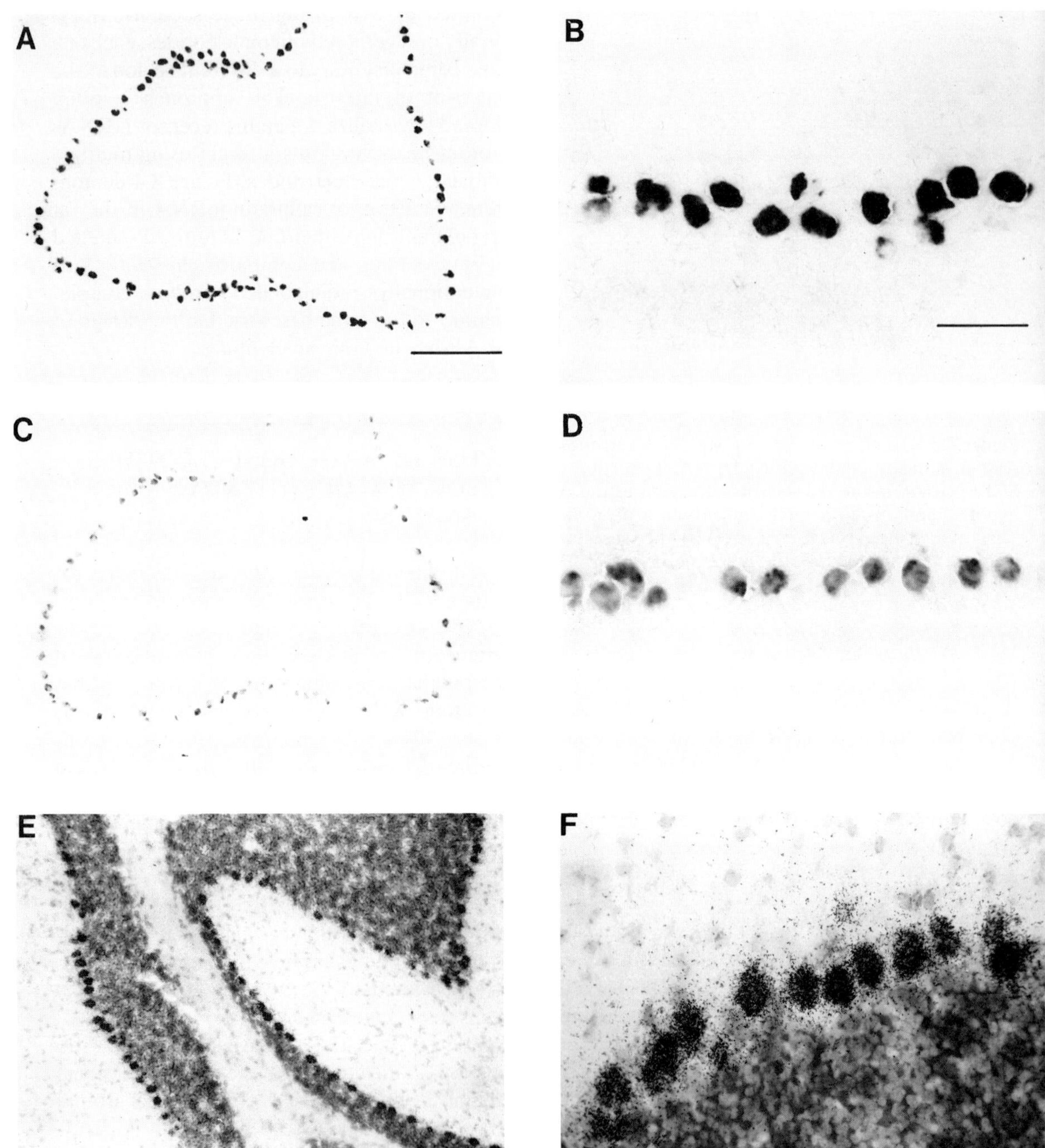

Figure 8.4 Expression of calbindin-D28K in the Purkinje cells of the rat cerebellum using multiple oligonucleotides. (A) and (B) Detection of calbindin transcripts using four AP-conjugated probes (kindly supplied by British Biotechnology); compare the intensity of the signal with (C) and (D), where only one oligonucleotide was used; sections were processed in parallel. The resolution and intensity of the signal in (A) and (B) compare favourably with the detection of calbindin message using conventional radioactive ISH techniques with four [α-[35S]thio]dATP- labelled calbindin oligonucleotides as shown in (E) and (F). (A), (C) and (E) were taken at the same magnification; scale bar = 100 μm (B), (D) and (F) are higher magnifications of the fields depicted in (A), (C) and (E) respectively.

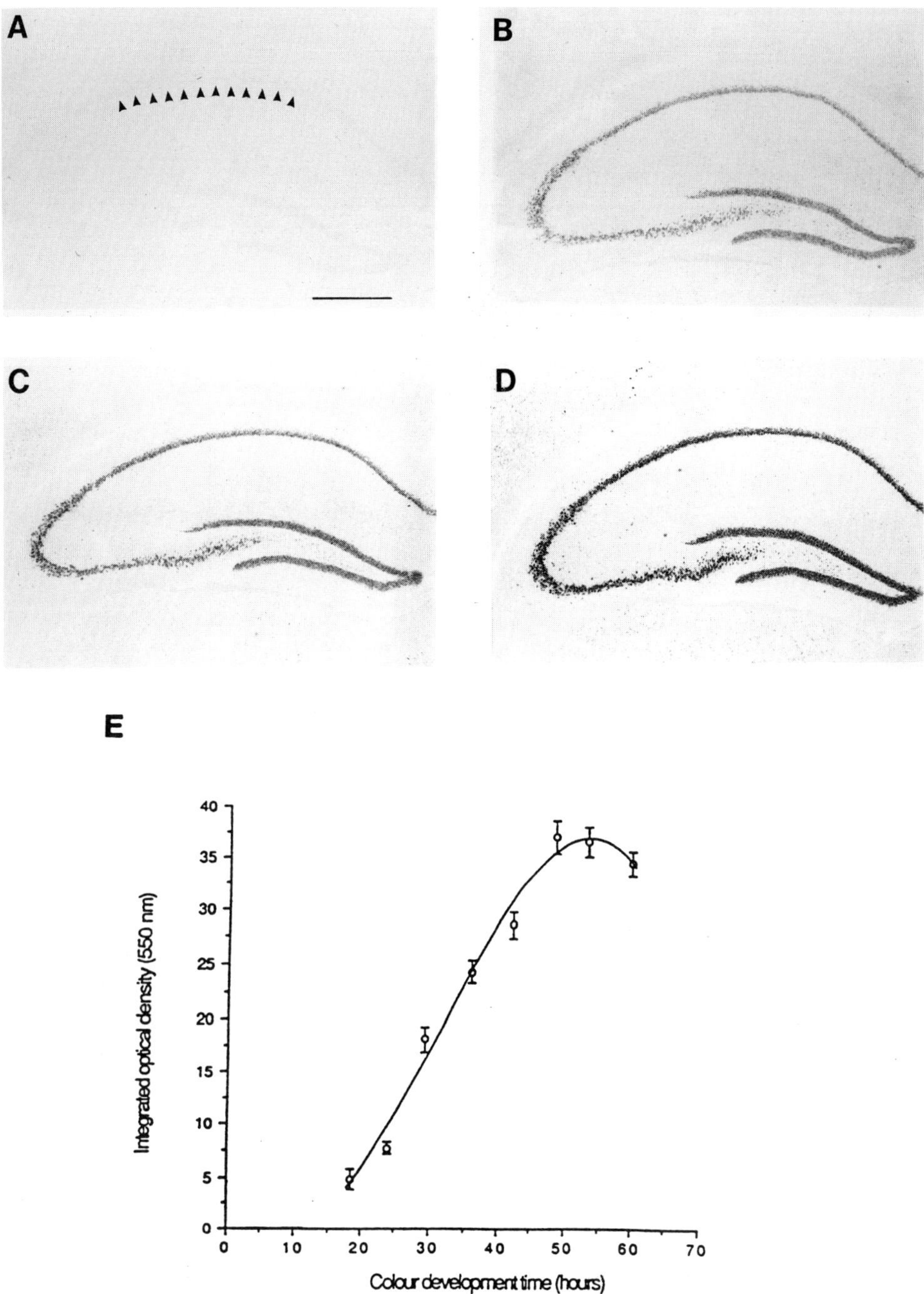

Figure 8.5 Colour-development time course profile for Ca^{2+}calmodulin kinase type II β (Cam-K II β) mRNA in the rodent hippocampus. The colour-development reaction was terminated at different time points, and the relative integrated optical density of the reaction product in the CA1 field of the hippocampus (indicated by arrows in A) was determined using a Vickers M85 microdensitometer. (A) 12 h development period, (B) 24 h development, (C) 36 h development, (D) 48 h development. (E) Graph showing the relationship between the density of the AP-reaction product in the pyramidal cells of the hippocampus (OD) and the colour-development time. The intensity of the hybridization signal increases linearly until ~48 h after which it begins to plateau. Scale bar = 250 μm.

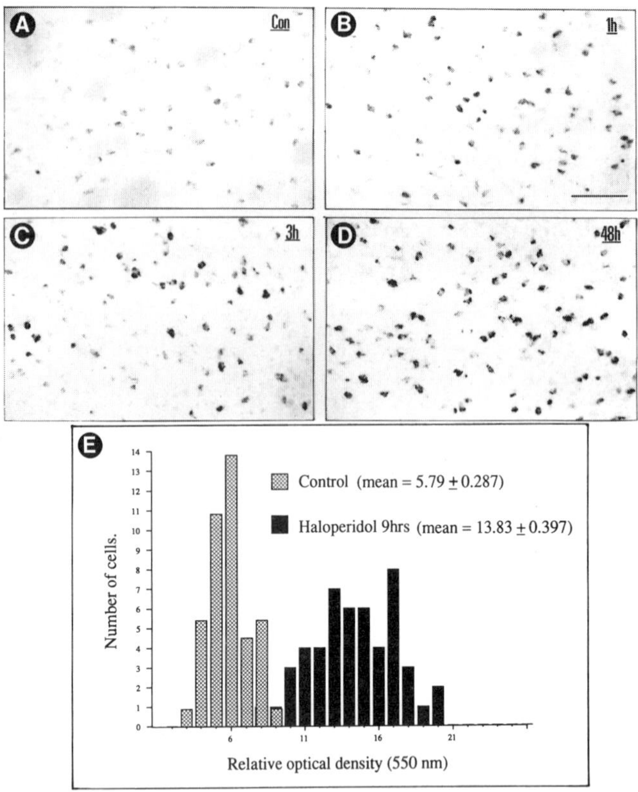

Figure 8.6 Rapid and sustained increase in enkephalin gene expression in the rat striatum after administration of the neuroleptic, haloperidol (4 mg kg^{-1}, i.p.). (A) control, (B) 1 h, (C) 3 h, (D) 48 h after injection of the drug. Note the increase in the cellular content of enkephalin mRNA within striatal cells. The bar graph in (E) demonstrates that the increase in enkephalin gene expression is reflected by a shift to the right in the integrated optical density per cell reflecting the increased cellular content of enkephalin mRNA. Scale bar = 100 μm. Reproduced with kind permission from Elsevier Science Publishers.

can be seen in Figure 8.6, an increase in the cellular content of pre-proenkephalin A mRNA in medium-sized striatal neurons after acute haloperidol administration is detected by the increased intensity of AP reaction product. It is important to note that all control and experimental sections are processed in parallel and that the colour-development time for all sections is the same.

Semiquantitative analysis of tissue sections hybridized with an AP-oligonucleotide may be carried out using a microdensitometer (Vickers M85) at 550 nm, the optimal wavelength for detecting AP reaction product using NBT and BCIP as substrates (Gutschmidt *et al.*, 1980). It is important to note that this type of analysis yields information about the relative changes in the *cellular* content of mRNA of interest. This is unlike film autoradiography (used for the analysis of a radioactive hybridization signal) where changes in optical density readings for an area of interest indicate changes in the mRNA content for that area. To establish if the changes in optical density measured off the autoradiograms reflect an increase in the cellular content of mRNA or/and an increase in the number of detectable cells expressing the mRNA of interest, sections must be processed for emulsion autoradiography so that silver deposits can indicate, using light microscopy, the cellular sites of hybridization.

8.6 SUITABLE CONTROLS FOR ISH

Problems associated with determining the 'ideal' ISH control are discussed in Chapter 1 (Section

1.7). We routinely hybridize 'control' sections with an excess of unlabelled oligonucleotide to demonstrate that the binding of the AP-oligonucleotide is displaceable. In addition, some sections are treated with RNAse before the hybridization stage to demonstrate that the probe is binding to single-stranded RNA (mRNA). Finally, Northern analysis is occasionally carried out using the cold oligonucleotide labelled with [^{32}P]dATP. Plotting a melting curve for each individual probe is sometimes carried out (by others) in an attempt to demonstrate the specificity of the hybridization signal; however, this is a tedious and time-consuming procedure.

8.7 COMBINING AP-OLIGONUCLEOTIDES AND [^{35}S]OLIGONUCLEOTIDES: COEXPRESSION STUDIES

For the simultaneous visualization of two mRNAs within a single neuron, we have developed a technique of coexpression (Kiyama *et al.*, 1991; Augood *et al.*, 1993) in which one mRNA is visualized using an AP-oligonucleotide and the other using an ^{35}S-labelled oligonucleotide. Ideally the two oligonucleotides used should be of similar length and GC content, so that the conditions of stringency for the two probes are similar. The least abundant mRNA should be detected using the radioactive probe, for example for the localization of dopamine (DA) receptor mRNAs and neuropeptide mRNAs in the rat basal ganglia, the DA receptor oligonucleotide would be radiolabelled with [α-[^{35}S]thio]dATP (see Chapter 1) and the neuropeptide oligonucleotide labelled with AP. Examples of coexpression are shown in Figures 8.7 and 8.8.

We have successfully demonstrated the cellular coexpression of two mRNAs in both fresh frozen cryostat sections and paraffin-embedded material (Kiyama *et al.*, 1991; Augood *et al.*, 1993; Emson *et al.*, 1993), illustrating further the versatility of this approach. Essentially, the standard hybridization protocol is followed (see Protocol 8.3 for fresh frozen sections and Protocol 8.4 for paraffin-embedded tissue) except that both the AP- and ^{35}S-labelled probes are diluted in the

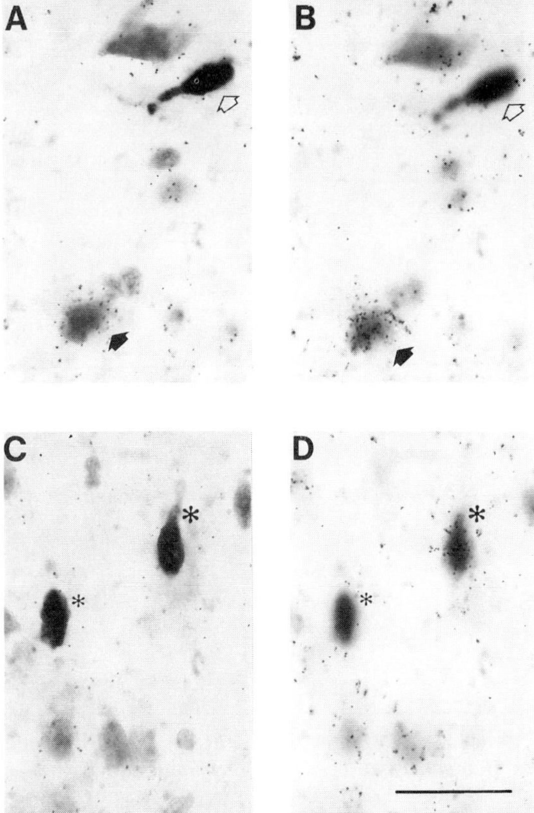

Figure 8.7 Coexpression of the AMPA receptor subunit, GluR2 mRNA and SRIF mRNA in the cerebral cortex. As noted in the text, clear and accurate photographic representation of coexpression studies can be difficult as the silver grains and AP reaction product are in different planes of focus. This is illustrated in (A) and (B) and (C) and (D) respectively. The same cortical field of view focused in (A) on the AP-reaction product (SRIF mRNA) and (B) on the silver grains (GluR2 mRNA), the neurone strongly expressing SRIF does not contain any GluR2 transcripts (open arrow) and the GluR2-expressing cell contains no AP-reaction product (closed arrow); the faint staining in the GluR2-expressing neuron is non-specific background. Similarly with (C) focused on AP-reaction product (SRIF mRNA) and (D) focused on silver grains (GluR2 mRNA), it can clearly be seen that one cortical neuron (large asterisk) contains both transcripts, and the other neuron (small asterisk) expresses only SRIF. Scale bar = 100 μm.

same hybridization buffer (with the addition of 3 μl ml^{-1} β-mercaptoethanol) and simultaneously applied to the fixed tissue section. Sections are then washed in 1×SSC at 55°C and processed for colour development as detailed in Protocol 8.5. Once the AP reaction product can be seen in the

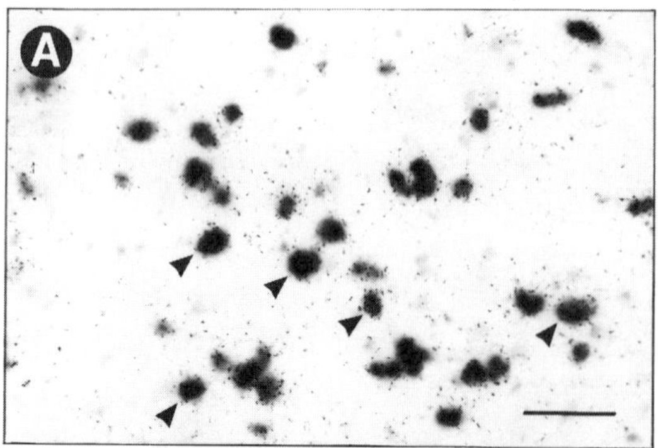

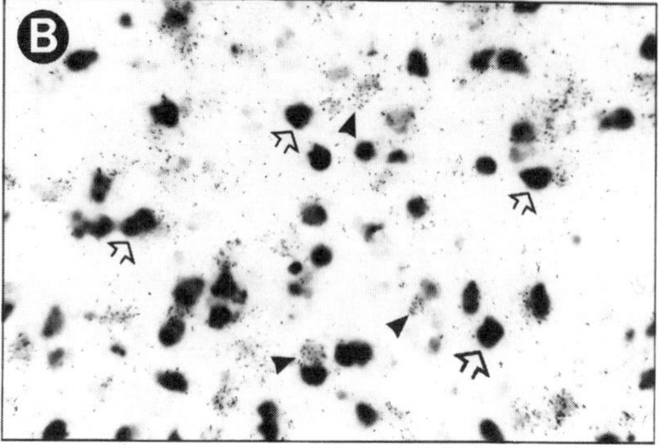

Figure 8.8 Cryostat sections of rat striatum hybridized simultaneously with (A) AP-enkephalin (ENK) probe and ^{35}S-labelled dopamine D_2 receptor oligonucleotide (silver grains), and (B) AP-ENK oligonucleotide and ^{35}S-labelled dopamine D_1 receptor oligonucleotide (silver grains). (A) Both hybridization signals (purple AP reaction product and silver grains) are concentrated within the same cells, indicating that ENK-expressing cells contain dopamine D_2 mRNA. Conversely in (B) the two hybridization signals appear concentrated in different cells illustrating that, in control rats, ENK (filled arrowheads) and dopamine D_1 receptor (open arrows) transcripts are not generally coexpressed. Scale bar = 50 μm. Reproduced with kind permission from Elsevier Science Publishers.

cytoplasm of positive cells, sections are washed extensively in Stop buffer, then rapidly dehydrated through a graded series of alcohol or acetone and processed for autoradiography (using Ilford K5 emulsion). For details of emulsion autoradiography refer to Chapter 1 (Protocol 1.9). After the desired exposure time to emulsion (routinely 4–14 weeks for neuropeptide/receptor mRNAs), sections should be developed and coverslipped with glycerin jelly. It is important to remember *not* to counterstain the sections. Using a light microscope the two hybridization signals can be

resolved easily; the coloured reaction product (corresponding to the AP-oligonucleotide) will be seen concentrated within the cell cytoplasm, and the silver grains, depicting sites where the ^{35}S-labelled oligonucleotide has hybridized, will be seen clustered over cells in a different plane of focus (see Figure 8.7). After colour development, to prevent non-specific discoloration of the tissue sections during the emulsion autoradiography stage, sections must be washed several times in Stop buffer. To aid visualization of both the radioactive and AP hybridization signals, we have found it best to stop the AP colour reaction before the mRNA-containing cells exhibit an intense colour signal, as this can sometimes mask the silver grain labelling, i.e. it is difficult to see black silver grains clustered over a cell containing a dark purple/black coloured reaction product. The reverse is also true: the silver grain labelling must not be so intense that the AP reaction product concentrated 'underneath' in the cell cytoplasm cannot be clearly seen. A compromise of hybridization signal intensity for both probes is ideal. Photographing the two signals to clearly illustrate the cellular coexpression of both hybridization signals is more difficult, if you cannot afford to publish in colour (see Figure 8.7)!!

8.8 COMBINING AP ISH AND IMMUNOCYTOCHEMISTRY

Although we have successfully combined AP ISH with immunocytochemistry on fresh frozen cryostat sections, paraffin-embedded material is the tissue of choice because of the excellent preservation of tissue morphology. As noted earlier, the order in which the two techniques are carried out can be critical if a good signal is to be obtained for both the ISH and immunocytochemistry. Although we generally perform the ISH step first and the immunocytochemistry second, there are examples when the immunocytochemistry must be performed first otherwise the antigen will be lost or denatured to such an extent (presumably by the formamide in the hybridization buffer) that it is not recognized by the antibody. This problem has been commented

Table 8.1 Problems encountered in AP hybridization.

Problem	Suggested reason and remedy
High AP background	Tissue sections dried out at some stage. High endogenous AP activity, e.g. in the intestine; treat sections with 0.2 M HCl for 10 min after fixation (see Protocol 8.3). AP-oligonucleotide too concentrated. Reduce [probe] BCIP stock soln should be clear, if coloured (brown) make up fresh stock.
No colour reaction	Was AP-probe added to HYB buffer? Check purity of ddH_2O; Milli-Q H_2O preferred for colour reaction. Check $MgCl_2$ concentration of Buffer B (see Section 8.4.1.2). Check that pH of Buffer B is between pH 9.0 and 9.5. Check activity of AP-oligonucleotide stock by spotting 0.5 µl of neat probe on a piece of filter paper, then add a drop of AP substrate solution (containing NBT and BCIP: see Protocol 8.5). The spot should go blue/purple within 1–3 min. No colour reaction suggests very low/no AP enzyme activity. Trying to detect a rare transcript; technique not sensitive enough. Try 3′-end labelling oligonucleotide with $[\alpha\text{-}[^{35}S]thio]dATP$ or use riboprobes.
Yellow crystals	Check temperature of colour development (20–25°C). Microfilter AP substrate solution just before use.
Low signal	Check through above pointers. Signal may be increased by mixing several AP-oligonucleotides together which are complementary to different regions of the transcript of interest (see Section 8.4.1.3). Signal to noise ratio may be increased by reducing the formamide concentration in the hybridization buffer from 50% to 40 or even 30% (to compensate for the inhibition of AP activity by formamide). Note of caution, this reduces the hybridization stringency.
High background after emulsion dipping	Sections not washed well enough in Stop buffer.

on in the literature by several authors (Schalling *et al.*, 1986; Shivers *et al.*, 1986; Watts & Swanson, 1989); indeed, for localization of oestrogen receptor immunoreactivity in the nucleus of hypothalamic cells, the antibody step must be carried out first using RNAse-free (DEPC-treated) solutions.

The protocol we use routinely involves carrying out the ISH step first (see Protocol 8.4), then, after detection of the AP reaction product, sections are rinsed extensively in Stop buffer and finally processed as detailed in Protocol 8.6. An example of the high quality of tissue morphology that can be obtained using paraffin-embedded tissue is given in Figures 8.1 and Colour Plate 2 which shows the co-localization of calretinin mRNA and calbindin immunoreactivity in cells of the substantia nigra.

8.9 TROUBLESHOOTING

Table 8.1 describes some problems encountered in AP hybridization and gives some reasons and remedies.

ACKNOWLEDGEMENTS

The authors would like to thank the MRC for financial support. N. Tønder and K. Westmore are thanked for their excellent technical assistance. EMM held a joint MRC-Merck Sharp & Dohme studentship.

Protocol 8.6 Combining ISH and immunocytochemistry.

(It is not necessary to use RNAse-free solutions for all the stages given below.)

1. First process sections for ISH using an AP-oligonucleotide (see Protocol 8.3 or 8.4).
2. After visualization of the AP reaction product, rinse tissue well in Stop buffer.
3. Rinse tissue for 10 min in 0.1 M PBS.
4. Incubate sections in 5% NGS[a] + 0.5% Triton X-100 in 0.1 M PBS to block non-specific binding.
5. Incubate sections in primary antibody diluted in PBS + 1% normal serum + 0.5% Triton X-100 for 24–48 h at 4°C. Sections may need to be overlaid with parafilm to prevent them from drying out.
6. Rinse sections for 5 × 10 min in PBS.
7. Incubate sections in horseradish peroxidase-conjugated goat anti-rabbit IgG[b] (1:500 for 2 h or 1:1000 overnight at 4°C). Alternatively use a Vector ABC kit and follow the manufacturer's instructions.
8. Wash sections for 5 × 10 min in PBS, then react with 0.05% DAB[c] activated with H_2O_2 (add 12 µl of 33% H_2O_2 to 100 ml of DAB solution).
9. Finally rinse sections well in an excess of PBS and coverslip using glycerin jelly.

[a] NGS, normal goat serum. Vary the species depending on the host of the IgG.
[b] Assuming the primary antibody was raised in rabbit, supplied by Vector.
[c] DAB, diaminobenzidine. This solution should be made up immediately before use.

REFERENCES

Agrawal, S., Christodoulou, C. & Gait, M.J. (1986) *Nucleic Acids Res.* **14**, 6227–6245.

Augood, S.J. & Emson, P.C. (1992) *Neuroscience* **47**, 317–324.

Augood, S.J., Kiyama, H., Faull, R.L.M. & Emson, P.C. (1991a) *Mol. Brain Res.* **9**, 341–346.

Augood, S.J., Kiyama, H., Faull, R.L.M. & Emson, P.C. (1991b) *Neuroscience* **44**, 35–44.

Augood, S.J., Faull, R.L.M. & Emson, P.C. (1992) *Eur. J. Neurosci.* **4**, 102–112.

Augood, S.J., Westmore, K., Faull, R.L.M. & Emson, P.C. (1993) *Mol Brain Res.* **20**, 328–334.

Brahic, M. & Haase, A.T. (1989) *Curr. Top. Microbiol. Immunol.* **143**, 9–20.

Emson, P.C. (1993) *Trends in Neuroscience* **16**, 9–16.

Emson, P.C., Heppelmann, B. & Augood, S.J. (1993) Development of techniques to combine isotopic and non-isotopic *in situ* hybridization, and immunocytochemistry for phenotypic character-ization of individual neurones. In *In situ hybrid-ization*, 2nd edn, J.D. Bardhas, K. Valentino & J. Eberwine (eds). Oxford University Press, Oxford, in press.

Finsen, B.R., Tønder, N., Augood, S. & Zimmer, J. (1992) *Neuroscience* **47**, 105–113.

Gähwiler, B.H. (1981) *J Neurosci Methods* **4**, 329–342.

Gähwiler, B.H. (1984) *Neuroscience* **11**, 751–760.

Gutschmidt, S., Lang, U. & Riecken, E.O. (1980). *Histochemistry* **69**, 189–202.

Heppelman, B., Señaris, R. & Emson, P.C. (1994) Combination of alkaline phosphatase *in situ* hybridization with immunohistochemistry: co-localization of calretinin-mRNA with calbindin and tyrosine hydroxylase immunoreactivity in rat substantia nigra neurones. *Brain Res.*, in press.

Hoefler, H., Childers, H., Montminy, M.R., Lechan, R.M., Goodman, R.H. & Wolfe, H.J. (1986) *Histochem. J.* **18**, 597–604.

Hopman, A.H.N., Wiegant, J., Tesser, G.I. & Van Duijin, P. (1986) *Nucleic Acids Res.* **14**, 6471–6488.

Jablonski, E., Moomaw, E.W., Tullis, R.H. & Ruth, J.L. (1986) *Nucleic Acids Res.* **14**, 6115–6128.

Kadowaki, K., McGowan, E.M., Mock, G., Chandler, S. & Emson, P.C. (1993) *Neurosci. Lett.* **153**, 80–84.

Kiyama, H. & Emson, P.C. (1990) *Neuroscience* **38**, 223–244.

Kiyama, H., Emson, P.C. & Ruth, J. (1990a) *Eur. J. Neurosci.* **2**, 512–524.

Kiyama, H., Emson, P.C., Ruth, J. & Morgan, C. (1990b) *Mol. Brain Res.* **7**, 213–219.

Kiyama, H., McGowan E. & Emson P.C. (1991) *Mol. Brain Res.* **9**, 87–93.

Langer, P.R., Waldrop, A.A. & Ward, D.C. (1981) *Proc. Natl. Acad. Sci. USA* **78**, 6633–6637.

Østergaard, K., Schou, J.P. & Zimmer, J. (1990) *Exp. Brain Res.* **82**, 547–565.

Østergaard, K., Schou, J.P., Gähwiler, B.H. & Zimmer, J. (1991) *Exp. Brain Res.* **83**, 357–365.

Pringle, J.H., Primrose, L., Kind, C.N., Talbot, I.C. & Launder, I. (1989) *J. Pathol.* **158**, 279–286.

Schalling, M., Hökfelt, T., Wallace, B., Goldstein, M., Filer, D., Yamin, C. & Schlesinger, D.H. (1986) *Proc. Natl. Acad. Sci. USA* **83**, 6208–6212.

Shivers, B.D., Harlan, R.E., Pfaff, D.W. & Schachter, B.S. (1986) *J. Histochem. Cytochem.* **34**, 39–43.

Watts, A.G. & Swanson, L.W. (1989) Combination of *in situ* hybridization with immunohistochemistry and retrograde tract tracing. In *Methods in neurosciences*, Vol. 1, P.M. Conn (ed.). Academic Press, London. pp. 127–136.

Wilkinson, D.G. (1992) The theory and practice of *in situ* hybridization. In *In situ hybridization, a practical approach*, D.G. Wilkinson (ed.) IRL Press, Oxford. pp. 1–13.

Wolber, R.A. & Lloyd, R.V. (1988) *Hum. Pathol.* **19**, 741–763.

CHAPTER NINE

Combining non-radioactive *in situ* hybridization with immunohistological and anatomical techniques

PETRA WAHLE

Lehrstuhl für Allg. Zoologie und Neurobiologie, Ruhr-Universität, ND 7/31, Postfach 10 21 48, D-44780 Bochum, Germany

9.1 INTRODUCTION

9.1.1 Why do we need to identify mRNA-expressing cell types?

In situ hybridization (ISH) allows us to localize in any given tissue the cells that express a particular gene. Because of the structural complexity of nervous tissue, we need to know in addition in which of the different neuronal (or glial) cell types the mRNA is expressed and in which functional circuits the cell type is involved? This information becomes very important in the light of recent discoveries that not only the functional but also the molecular features of neurons are maintained and can be modified by activity-dependent mechanisms. Analysis of trans-synaptic regulation of gene expression in a complex neuronal network requires the localization of mRNA and the concurrent characterization of molecular, morphological and anatomical features. Any ISH protocol employed must therefore meet these requirements. Further, in this work we are analysing the developing CNS, and we have to deal with very fragile tissue. A method is therefore needed that preserves its structural integrity.

9.1.2 Why use non-radioactive cRNA probes?

This chapter describes a method of ISH using digoxigenin (DIG)-UTP-labelled cRNA probes. The DIG molecule is a unique steroid isolated from the plant *Digitalis purpurea*. Linked to UTP, it can be incorporated as a marker into cRNA probes. Specific antibodies against DIG allow the subsequent detection of the DIG-labelled probes. The reasons for employing non-radioactive methods are obvious and have been discussed previously (see Emson (1993) for a recent review): radioactive isotopes, which are expensive to buy and dispose of, are not required; radioactive waste is not produced;

IN SITU HYBRIDIZATION PROTOCOLS FOR THE BRAIN
ISBN 0–12–759919–3

there is no need for a special laboratory with extra equipment for making and storing probes, performing experiments and developing the material (isotope laboratory darkrooms); there is no radiation risk to personnel and the environment.

Further, DIG-labelled probes are stable for months, as they have no physically decaying tag. cRNA probes, however, are synthetic RNA and are thus more sensitive to degradation than DNA oligonucleotides. To protect the probe, gloves must be worn throughout the hybridization, and equipment has to be as clean as possible and RNAse-free. Once this becomes routine, however, riboprobes are as at least as easy to handle as radioactive probes.

When a cloned sequence cannot be obtained, it is of course an advantage to design a probe according to the published sequence and order oligonucleotides from a service laboratory, so that only a labelling reaction has to be carried out (see Chapter 1).

In contrast, to prepare the cRNA probe, one needs the template DNA, usually cloned into a plasmid (transcription vector). To produce the template and the probe further requires the basic equipment of a molecular biology laboratory and technical know-how. However, cRNA probes offer several advantages. An *in vitro* transcription yields enough probe for a series of experiments. Further, when DIG-UTP is used as a marker the transcribed probe is stable for months, which is advantageous for a developmental study for example, and the variable 'probe activity' can be excluded. Further, the RNA polymerases synthesizing the probes are highly specific for their promoter, thereby generating either antisense (complementary to cellular mRNA) or (a suitable control) sense (same as cellular mRNA) probes. Non-raioactive probes are detected immunologically. The methods are straightforward and standard in many laboratories, as is enzyme-based colorimetric detection. The procedure is short; it can be carried out within 2–3 days. Signal development can be controlled by eye (microscope). The hybridized tissue can be directly processed for detection of additional markers.

9.1.3 Organization of this chapter

The chapter is organized in the order that an experiment would be carried out, starting with probe preparation, tissue preparation, the hybridization and subsequent detection of cell type-specific markers. At the end of Sections 9.4, 9.5, 9.6 and 9.7, the staining results are described and discussed. They have been obtained in recent experiments. At the end of every section, recipes are given for the buffers and solutions, and a list of the equipment used in our laboratory. Molecular biological techniques not directly related to the topic of the article may be acquired from *Current Protocols in Molecular Biology (CPMB)* (Ausubel *et al.*, 1987) or Sambrook *et al.*, 1987.

9.2 THE PROBES

9.2.1 Preparation of plasmid DNA for transcription

The sequences were obtained from the colleagues mentioned in the Acknowledgements. The sequences were either already inserted into transcription vectors, or fragments of interest were subcloned by us and transformed into appropriate bacteria (CPBM, Chapter 1.8). Once a clone had been obtained and characterized, a 100 ml culture was grown (CPBM, Chapter 1.7). Plasmid DNA was isolated on anion-exchange 'Qiagen' columns Pack-100 (Quiagen, USA; Diagen, Germany). The kit comes with the buffers and a detailed protocol, and yields a high amount of pure plasmid DNA.

About 10 μg of the DNA was digested with restriction enzymes cutting downstream of promoter and insert (CPMB, Chapter 3). Linearized DNA was purified with phenol/chloroform and with precipitated ethanol (CPMB, Chapter 2.1), which removes proteins and desalts the DNA. Gloves, sterile equipment and RNA-grade chemicals must be used. RNA polymerases and the riboprobes are very sensitive to contamination, and care must be

Protocol 9.1

1. To 1 µg of template dissolved in 13 µl of water on ice add
   2 µl of 10× transcription buffer
   2 µl of 10× nucleic acid-labelling mixture
   2 µl (20–40 units) of RNA polymerase
2. Vortex briefly and spin down to bottom of the tube.
3. Incubate at 37°C for 2 h.
4. Add 10–20 units of an RNAase-free DNAase, to digest the template DNA. Mix.
5. Incubate at 37°C for 15 min.
6. Add 1 µl of 0.5 M EDTA, pH 8.0 (DEPC-treated!) to stop the reaction. Mix.
7. Precipitate the labelled RNA with 0.1 vol. of 4 M LiCl and 3 vol. of ice-cold ethanol.
8. Leave at −70°C for 30 min.
9. Pellet the RNA by centrifugation at 14 000 **g** for 30 min.
10. Pour off supernatant and wash pellet with 50 µl of 80% ethanol. A large brownish pellet, often somewhat fuzzy, should be obtained.
11. Remove the ethanol with a pipette.
12. Cover tube opening and inner lid with a piece of parafilm (the unexposed side). Poke in a tiny hole with sterile needle.
13. Dry the pellet in a speed-vac. The parafilm protects the RNA.
14. Dissolve pellet in 90 µl of DEPC-treated water at 37°C for 30 min. Make sure water, tubes and pipette tips are RNAase-free. Vortex or pipette up and down.
15. When dissolved, take 2 µl into a separate tube.
16. To the rest add 10 µl of 10× TER (100 mM Tris/HCl, pH 7.5, 50 mM EDTA, pH 8.0, 1 mg ml^{-1} yeast tRNA). Mix. An RNAase inhibitor may be added to 50 units ml^{-1}.
17. Store the riboprobe at −20°C.

taken to ensure that the template DNA is pure. After the precipitation, the DNA pellet was washed with 80% ethanol (made with DEPC-treated water) and dried in a speed-vac.

DNA was dissolved in 20 µl of RNAase-free water (pure double-distilled water; we used water from a Millipore unit, treated with DEPC and autoclaved twice). Then 1 µl was run together with a standard DNA of known concentration on an agarose gel stained with ethidium bromide to determine the concentration (CPBM, Chapter 2.5). The linearized template should appear as a single sharp band of the predicted size. About 1 µg was taken in 10 µl of water for the transcription reaction. It was allowed to stand for 30 min on ice to ensure that the DNA was completely dissolved (it was slowly pipetted up and down several times with sterile RNAase-free pipette tips or vortexed carefully).

9.2.2 *In vitro* transcription

Gloves, sterile equipment and RNA-grade chemicals should be used. Riboprobes are synthesized with the nucleic acid (RNA) labelling kit (no. 1175025; Boehringer, Mannheim, Germany). It contains a 10× transcription buffer, RNA polymerases (SP6/T7 or T3 T7 at 20 units µl^{-1}) and a 10× acid mixture containing the (DIG)-labelled UTP (10 mM ATP, CTP, GTP; 65. mM UTP and 3.5 mM DIG-UTP). Buffers and polymerases from other companies work well too. An RNAase inhibitor may be included in the reaction mixture, but is not necessary if reagents are RNAase-free. The reaction volume is 20 µl.

9.2.3 How to check transcription efficiency and quality of the probes

There are basically two reasons for failure of the procedure. One is probe quality. Newly

Protocol 9.2

1. Take 1 µl of control RNA.
2. Heat-denature at 65°C for about 5 min.
3. Mix it with an equal volume (1 µl) of methylmercury hydroxide (MeHgOH, from Serva) containing loading buffer (see the chapter on gel electrophoresis of RNA in Maniatis *et al.* (1992)). Note, that MeHgOH is very toxic, so work in a fume hood).
4. Heat 2 µl of the labelled RNA dissolved in water to denature, and mix with 2 µl of MeHgOH. Store samples on ice.
5. Prepare a minigel. Take a glass plate (e.g. 5 cm × 7.5 cm) or large glass slide that fits into a minigel chamber and a comb. Clean equipment by rinsing in 1% SDS/water, followed by sterile water. Dry comb and glass plate by a rinse in technical-grade ethanol. Mount comb 0.5–1 mm above the glass plate with two gel clamps on a level bench.
6. Dissolve RNA-grade agarose in 1× borate buffer. Allow to cool to 55°C.
7. Add ethidium bromide to 0.2 µg ml^{-1}.
9. Pipette, with a baked-glass pipette, 10 ml of agarose on top of the glass plate. Surface tension keeps the solution on the glass, and it solidifies quickly. The comb forms shallow slots. Mount gel into chamber, fill with borate buffer.
10. Carefully load the RNA samples (the slots take up to 5 µl), and run the gel in 1× borate buffer at 50 V.
11. Visualize bands under UV light.
12. Perform a Northern blot (CPBM, Chapter 4.9) with the gel. Transfer in 20 × SSC for at least 4 h on to nylon membrane (Hybond N, Amersham).
13. UV cross-link the RNA to the membrane (2–3 min, or fix by baking for 2 h at 80°C in vacuum oven.

The following steps are not performed under sterile conditions. The buffer recipes are given at the end of the chapter.

14. Rinse the membrane 2 × 2 min in distilled water, then for 2 × 5 min in buffer DIG-I.
15. Block with 5% bovine serum albumin (BSA; fraction V) in buffer DIG-I, or blocking reagent (Boehringer) diluted in DIG-I for 30 min at room temperature.
16. Briefly rinse off blocking solution and incubate membrane in anti-DIG antibody (sheep F(ab)$_2$ fragments; Boehringer) tagged with alkaline phosphatase (AP) diluted 1:5000 in DIG-I for 1 h at room temperature.
17. Rinse in DIG-I for 3 × 10 min.
18. Equilibrate for 2–3 min in two changes of TBS/Mg^{2+} buffer, pH 9.5.
19. Incubate in substrate solution in TBS/Mg^{2+} buffer using nitroblue tetrazolium (NBT) and X-phosphate (5-bromo-4-chloro-3-indolyl phosphate; BCIP). For the incubations, membranes are heat-sealed into plastic bags. Volumes should be kept as low as possible for a 5 × 7.5 cm membrane use 5 ml of solution). Signals should develop within 2 h. Stop the reaction in water after the bands have appeared. Allow filter to dry.
20. The labelled RNA should appear as a more or less sharp band.

synthesized probes should be checked by gel electrophoresis and Northern blotting. To generate good-quality probes general molecular biological techniques and rules for maintaining an RNAase-free environment should be followed. Gloves, sterile equipment and RNA-grade chemicals should be used. To check the cRNA, a labelled RNA of known size (760 bp) and

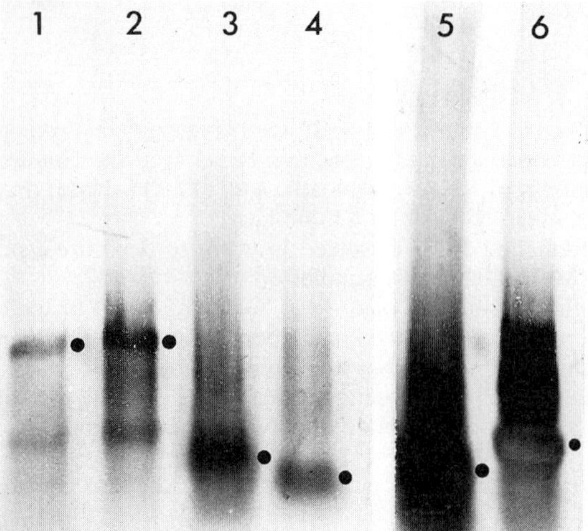

Figure 9.1 Northern blot of a minigel reveals *in vitro* transcribed cRNA probes labelled with DIG-UTP. Lane 1, 2.3 kb GAD antisense cRNA; lane 2, 2.3 kb GAD sense cRNA; lane 3, 0.4 kb NPY exon 2 antisense; lane 4, 0.28 kb NPY signal peptide antisense; lane 5, 0.34 kb β-preprotachykinin exons 1–4 antisense; lane 6, 0.76 kb DIG-labelled control RNA. Major bands are indicated by dots. Note, that bands have different intensities as a result of different transcription efficiencies. The major band in lane 6 is so overloaded that owing to steric hindrance of antibody, it appears less well stained than the rest. Lanes 1 and 2 have partial transcripts running below the expected cRNA size. This occurs sometimes, but has no effect on ISH results.

concentration 100 ng μl^{-1}) which comes with the Boehringer RNA-labelling kit can be used.

Results are shown in Figure 9.1. These cRNAs had been dissolved in 100 μl, and 1 μl was run on the gel. Transcripts from different templates are shown. The size of the transcripts can be determined using the control RNA band of 760 bp. The concentration can be judged by comparing the staining intensity of the bands. The control probe was very concentrated, and was not effectively denatured. Multiple bands appear. Lane 5 is overloaded too. The transcription yielded a very high amount of probe. Transcription was less efficient for probes run in lanes 1–4, but all yielded good ISH results at an appropriate dilution (see Section 9.4.1). A smear below a band indicates partial transcripts. Such probes may still be used for ISH. Degraded probes may run as a smear with no band of the expected size.

The absence of bands indicates failure of transcription; this can usually already be seen after precipitation of the transcription reaction (no pellet). Reasons may be impurities of template DNA, badly dissolved DNA, wrong concentration of buffer or RNAase contamination of ingredients or equipment (see CPBM for troubleshooting transcription reactions).

9.2.4 Storage of probes

We store labelled RNA at −20°C in aliquots of 20–30 μl. Repeated freeze-thaw does not change probe quality. Probes should be thawed in the hand or in a 37°C waterbath. If RNAase inhibitor is included, the probe should not be thawed at 65°C, because this inactivates the inhibitor and may release bound RNAases. Probes are vortexed before use. There should be no precipitate. We are currently using probes synthesized more than 8 months ago, and probe quality has remained unchanged.

9.3 THE TISSUE

ISH on different kinds of 'brain tissue' is presented in this Chapter, namely rat and cat brain, organotypic cultures of rat visual cortex grown on coverslips by the roller-tube technique, and dissociated cultures of rat hypothalamic neurons grown in cell culture dishes. Brain tissue is usually fixed by perfusion.

9.3.1 Fixation by perfusion

Animal brain tissue is optimally fixed by vascular perfusion of a physiological salt solution followed by the fixative (see also CPMB, Chapter 14). The salt solution rinses out the blood, so that it does not clog blood vessels and allows the fixative to reach the capillaries.

The solutions are in glass bottles with an outlet placed about 1 m above the animal. The bottles are connected with tubing to a T-shaped adaptor. Stop cocks are placed in the tubing to start and

Protocol 9.3

Equipment: gel chamber, plates, combs, clamps, power supply, nylon membrane (Amersham Hybond N), UV light table 302 nm, polaroid camera, microlitre pipettes, sterile Eppendorf tubes and tips.

Reagents: agarose (RNA-grade), technical-grade ethanol, restriction enzymes (New England Biolabs; buffers included), blocking reagent and sheep anti-DIG labelled with AP (F(ab)$_2$-fragments).

Solutions:

DEPC-treated water: Per litre of double-distilled water (e.g. from a Millipore unit) in a baked glass flask add under a fume hood 1 ml of DEPC (Sigma Chemicals, St. Louis, MO, USA). Stir for at least 30 min, until the oily substance is dispersed. Autoclave twice.

5× buffer DIG-I: 121 g of Tris/HCl and 87.6 g of NaCl dissolved in 1260 ml of double-distilled water. Add 740 ml of 1 M HCl to pH 7.5. Autoclave. Dilute to 1× with distilled water. The 1× buffer does not need to be autoclaved.

1× TBS/Mg^{2+} buffer pH 9–9.5: 100 ml of 1 M Tris base, brought to pH 9.5 with about 25 ml of 1 NHCl; then add 20 ml of 5 M NaCl to 950 ml of double distilled water. Add 50 ml of 1 M MgCl$_2$. Mix and use.

MeHgOH solution: Mix in a fume hood 4.75 ml of DEPC-treated water with 1 ml of 10× borate buffer (final concentration 1×), 0.25 ml of 1 M MeHgOH (Serva; final concentration 25 mM), 2 ml of glycerol (final concentration 20%), 2 ml of 1% Bromophenol Blue (final concentration 0.2%). Divide into 1 ml portions and store frozen. To use, mix 1:1 with the heat-denatured (10 min 65°C) RNA sample and load on an agarose/borate gel.

10× borate buffer: 30.09 g of boric acid (0.5 M), 19.10 g of sodium tetraborate, 10 H$_2$O (0.05 M), 14.2 g of sodium sulphate (0.1 M) add 1 litre of double-distilled water. Add 1 ml of DEPC, stir, autoclave.

Ethidium bromide stock: 10 mg ml^{-1} sterile water. Carcinogenic! Use 10 μl per 100 ml of agarose solution.

20× SSC: 3 M NaCl, 0.3 M sodium citrate in double-distilled water. Treat with DEPC, autoclave twice.

EDTA: 0.5 M dissolves when pH reaches 8.0. Treat with DEPC, autoclave twice. Make up small amount, aliquot and freeze.

LiCl: 4 M, treat with DEPC, autoclave twice. Make up small amount, aliquot and freeze.

AP substrates: NBT is 75 mg ml^{-1} in 70% (v/v) dimethylformamide. Store aliquots at −20°C. BCIP is 50 mg ml^{-1} in dimethylformamide. Store at −20°C. Both substances are included in the nucleic acid detection kit (Boehringer), but can also be made up with reagents from other companies. We usually have 2 ml of each in the freezer.

Other chromogenes for AP: a red reaction product is yielded with Fast Violet B (final concentration 0.2 mg ml^{-1}) and Naphthol-AS-E-phosphate (final concentration 0.1 mg ml^{-1}), both from Serva. The combination may be used for histological detection (Chapter 4).

---

stop the flow and to regulate the flow rate. The adaptor's third arm connects to the perfusion cannula with a piece of tubing that is smaller in diameter. Instead of a cannula, a piece of tubing (diameter approximately the size of the arterial stem) can be inserted into the heart. The cannula is filled to the tip with salt solution, but there must not be fixative in the first flush. Solutions do not need to be autoclaved.

Fixatives: We use freshly made 4% para-

Protocol 9.4

1. Deeply anaesthetize the animal by intraperitoneal injection of pentobarbitone (Nembutal; 60 mg kg^{-1} body weight is a lethal overdose).
2. Wait until reflexes and breathing have stopped (pinch the toes, or touch the cornea of the eye).
3. Open the thorax with large scissors (the lungs will collapse).
4. Carefully open the pericard (fine scissors), and steady the heart with a pair of forceps by gripping the right ventricle.
5. Poke a hole the size of the perfusion cannula into the left ventricle (use sharp tip of fine scissors to penetrate the muscle).
6. Take care not to disrupt the septum. Aim towards the left ventricle.
7. Carefully insert the cannula filled to the tip with 0.9% NaCl in 50 mM sodium phosphate buffer, pH 7.5, or commercial Ringer's solution in distilled water.
8. Cut open the right atrium (avoid cutting other parts of the heart or arterial stem) and start the perfusion. Blood should start flowing out of the right atrium. There should be no leakage out of the left ventricle (backflow occurs if the cut is larger than the cannula) or out of the nostrils/snout (this happens when the septum is penetrated or perfusion pressure is too high, in which case immediately reduce the flow rate).
9. Wait about half a minute (for rat; wait longer, if a bigger animal is perfused) until the solution flowing out of right atrium starts to become clear.
10. Close, with the stop cock, the flow of saline, and open the flow of fixative. The body will show a muscular tremor, the limbs will stretch, and neck and limbs will stiffen, when the fixative reaches the muscles. This indicates a good perfusion. Perfuse about 200–400 ml of fixative per rat.

formaldehyde which gives the best retention of cellular RNA. Use ice-cold, if this is required for subsequent immunohistological procedures. Use additives, if required for detection of antigens e.g. glutardialdehyde is required for detection of amino acid transmitters. The concentration should be kept as low as possible. The ISH procedure in sections tolerates 0.2% glutardialdehyde. Picric acid was found to improve fixation of very immature tissue. The ISH procedure tolerates 1% picric acid. Other fixatives have not been tried in our laboratory. It is not necessary to add DEPC. Also, never autoclave fixatives!

Tissue is dissected out of the skull and dropped into fixative. Use gloves and clean equipment now to handle the tissue. The block containing the structure of interest is dissected from the brain and rinsed in fixative. With fine forceps remove the dura and pia mater. Rinse tissue block in several changes of fixative. The block may be stored for several hours at +4°C in fixative (4% paraformaldehyde) to postfix. Postfixation time depends on the quality of the perfusion. Also, some antigens require longer fixation; this has to be determined empirically.

Organotypic 'roller tube' cultures are prepared as described (Gähwiler, 1988). To harvest cultures for ISH, briefly rinse off medium in sterile 100 mM sodium phosphate buffer pH 7.5, or with Hank's balanced salt solution (Gibco). Fix with cold 4% phosphate-buffered paraformaldehyde for 30–60 min. Do not use glutardialdehyde if whole-mount cultures are to be processed. The culture technique requires tissue embedding in a plasma–thrombin clot, which is hard to remove without destroying the tissue. Glutardialdehyde-containing fixatives apparently cause the plasma–thrombin clot and/ or the glia layer that surrounds the tissue to become impenetrable for probes.

Dissociated neuronal cultures of embryonic rat

hypothalamus are prepared as described and grown in 35-mm cell culture dishes on a glia feeder layer (Swandulla & Misgeld, 1990). Cultures are rinsed with sterile PBS (0.1 M sodium phosphate, 0.9% NaCl) and fixed with 4% buffered paraformaldehyde at 4°C for 30 min.

9.3.2 Preparation of sections

After the fixation, the tissue block has to be cryoprotected before freeze cutting. For a rat brain, 100 ml of cryoprotection solution is prepared. The tissue is placed in a sterile beaker, and rinsed with 2 × 5 ml of cryoprotection solution. The tissue block is transferred into cryoprotection solution and left overnight at +4°C. Next morning the block will have sunk to the bottom of the beaker. This indicates complete immersion in sucrose. The block can now be frozen.

The tissue block is frozen from base to top on dry ice in a small puddle of TissueTek (OTC compound, Miles) or other type of cryomounting medium. A fresh bottle is reserved for freezing tissue for ISH. During freezing, the block is completely surrounded with the cryomedium. Alternatively, the tissue is frozen directly on to the chuck in a −40°C cryostat and equilibrated to the cutting temperature (−15 to −20°C) for about 15 min.

Meanwhile, the equipment is set up to cut and collect the sections. A normal cryostat knife (C-knife) is used, gloves being used for handling. Usually, knifes are oiled after use to prevent corrosion. The knife should be cleaned with 1% SDS, rinsed in distilled water and dried by a rinse in ethanol. When dry, it is inserted into the cryostat and allowed to cool. To transfer sections, we use glass hooks bent and polished over a bunsen burner flame from Pasteur pipettes baked overnight at 180°C. The hooks are then wrapped in aluminium foil. Sterile baked glass Petri dishes are used to collect the cryostat sections. The first dish can be filled with 2 × SSC to dissolve the cryomedium and the second dish with a mixture of 2 × SSC and hybridization solution. This allows stepwise equilibration of sections to the hybridization solution. In the case of proteinase K (PK), for which pretreatment of sections is required for detection of low-level mRNAs, a further Petri dish is required. It is filled with PK buffer (100 mM Tris/HCl, pH 8.0, 50 mM EDTA and PK to 1–2 µg ml^{-1}) and placed on a small hot plate maintained at 37°C. Sections are collected directly into PK solution and incubated for 15–30 min for digestion. The incubation time for each section must be noted. The section is then transferred to the dish filled with 2 × SSC, then to 2 × SSC/hybridization solution.

For the incubations we use 30-well glass plates (about 17 cm × 20 cm; the wells are 2.5 cm in diameter and 2 mm deep) covered with a glass lid. Their advantage is they can be easily cleaned, wrapped in aluminium foil and baked at 180°C overnight and may be reused many times. When large series of sections are to be processed (Wahle *et al.* (1993) processed for each experiment about 180 serial sections of the adult cat midbrain and thalamus at a time), cell culture plates (e.g. 36-well plates) can be used. If it is not important to have serial sections, one may collect and incubate several sections in a small glass vial (5–10 ml in volume). This works well for immunohistochemistry and we have tried it successfully for ISH.

Sections are cut at a thickness of 20–60 µm. Section thickness depends on the type of experiment and also on the quality of fixation. Well-fixed material, or older developmental stages, or adult animals, or material for double-labelling experiments are usually cut at 20–30 µm. Immature tissue (e.g. newborn cat cortex) is very fragile, and thicker sections survive the procedure much better. We have successfully hybridized sections as thick as 75 µm. Generally, the better the sections the better the results of the hybridization. Sections should be cut at low speed.

We have also tried successfully vibratome sections for semithin plastic embedding described earlier (Wahle & Beckh, 1992). The equipment should be cleaned with 1% SDS followed by sterile water. Ethanol is used to dry equipment if necessary. The tissue is mounted on a sterile chuck with HistoAcryl or cyan-based glue. Sections are cut under sterile phosphate buffer.

9.3.3 Tissue culture systems

Organotypic cultures are usually hybridized *in toto*. Fixative is rinsed off in three changes (10 ml each) of 2 × SSC. The coverslips are then removed from the culture tubes with blunt forceps. The plasma clot is scraped away as well as possible with a scalpel. The tissue is then taken from the coverslips with a scalpel or razor, and floated onto 2 × SSC/prehybridization solution, and transferred with glass hooks to prehybridization solution in a glass well plate.

Dissociated cultures are rinsed with 2 × SSC to remove the fixative, followed by a mixture of 2 × SSC/prehybridization mix, followed by 0.6 ml of prehybridization mix per small dish. Cultures are prehybridized for 4 h at the desired temperature.

9.3.4 Storage of tissue and sections

Tissue frozen as described above can be wrapped in aluminium foil and stored for months at −70°C. For use, it must be removed from this temperature, the foil peeled away, and the tissue mounted on a chuck and equilibrated to the cutting temperature in the cryostat (at least 30 min). Also, a block under investigation can be stored at −70°C and may be reused later. The block must be completely covered with cryomedium; this is necessary to prevent drying of the tissue. It is then wrapped in foil and left at −70°C.

Sections, once cut, may be stored at −20°C in hybridization solution in small glass vials covered with parafilm or in Eppendorf tubes (few small sections per tube) or in 15 ml polypropylene tubes (larger sections). For some experiments it is necessary to cut several series of alternating sections. One or two are hybridized immediately, the other series are well equilibrated to hybridization solution, transferred to an appropriate tube and stored at −20°C. For hybridization, a series of sections are simply warmed up to room temperature and transferred separately into well plates with fresh hybridization solution. In this way 'aliquots' of sections can be maintained

Protocol 9.5

Equipment: baked glass vials, glass well plates and Petri dishes, aluminium foil, cryostat, C-knife, 1% SDS, technical-grade ethanol, Pasteur pipettes, Eppendorf pipettes, sterile tubes and tips, hybridization oven.

Reagents: molecular-biology-grade (or highest purity) chemicals for the solutions.

Solutions:

Paraformaldehyde 4%: Dissolve 40 g in 300 ml of distilled water brought to 70°C (chemical hood) with a few drops of 1 M NaOH. The milky solution should clear immediately. Reduce heat. Buffer with sodium phosphate to pH 7.5 and 100 mM final concentration; it is best to add 0.5 vol. of buffer from a 2× stock solution. Make up with distilled water to 1000 ml. Filter and allow to cool to room temperature. Add additives.

Cryoprotection solution: 20% sucrose (RNAase-free reagent) dissolved in DEPC-treated 100 mM sodium phosphate, pH 7.5. Do not treat sucrose solution with DEPC and do not autoclave.

Prehybridization solution: 50% formamide (Fluka or Baker, deionized), 250 µg ml^{-1} heat-denatured and sheared salmon sperm DNA, 100 µg ml^{-1} yeast tRNA, 0.05 M sodium phosphate buffer, pH 6.5, 4 × SSC, 5% dextran sulphate, 0.02% BSA, 0.02% polyvinylpyrrolidone, 0.02% Ficoll 400. We usually make 500 ml or so, having the ingredients as stock solutions. The mix is then divided into 15 ml portions and stored at −20°C. To thaw, bring to 65°C, and vortex to completely dissolve any whitish precipitate. When adding probe, vortex vigorously to ensure complete mixing.

either to be included in an experiment as a positive control or to quickly test newly synthesized probes. I have obtained normal results on material stored for up to 4 months so far. Also, there is no loss of mRNA or antigenicity. A hybridization buffer contains more or less the same ingredients (just more expensive) as solutions used to infiltrate tissue for long-term storage at −20°C in a non-frozen state.

Organotypic cultures are also stored prehybridized in Eppendorf tubes at −20°C. In this way *in vitro* cultures of different age or maintained under different culture conditions can be collected over a period of time to be hybridized concurrently later. This is more efficient and helps reduce experimental variability.

9.3.5 Troubleshooting tissue quality

A major reason for failure of the ISH procedure is poor tissue quality. There are several reasons why tissue may look poor. (1) It is not adequately fixed. It needs some expertise to perfuse an animal in order to obtain an optimally fixed brain. Try to keep surgery time within a few minutes to get access to the cardiovascular system as fast as possible. It is best to start the flow of saline when the heart is still beating. Take care to remove air bubbles from the tubing, as they may clog arteries. When dissecting the brain, try not to squeeze the tissue. (2) When perfusion pressure is too high, blood vessels may disrupt, and cell membranes too. The morphology is destroyed, and worse, RNAases gain access to cellular mRNA. Under the microscope, such tissue has a lot of holes, and ISH reaction product, if present, is not confined to cell bodies. Try to lower the bottles with fixative, reduce flow rate of solutions, try smaller perfusion cannulas. (3) Cryoprotection is not adequate. This results in freezing artefacts (shatter, cracks). Allow more time to immerse the block in sucrose. It must be sunk to the bottom of the container (through at least 5 cm of sucrose cushion). Time depends on block size. (4) Freezing the tissue may cause artefacts. Try to blot away excess sucrose and cover block (on a piece of sterile aluminium foil) with TissueTek. Then mount block with its base in TissueTek on a cryostat

chuck and allow to freeze from bottom to top. Then cover block completely with TissueTek, but avoid thawing/refreezing of the surface. It will give cracks in the sections. Avoid air bubbles in the TissueTek. (5) Cryostat cutting needs expertise. Artefacts are often breaks parallel to the knife, because tissue is too cold. Allow time to equilibrate to a higher temperature. We usually cut with a block temperature of −15 to −20°C, and chamber temperature set to −30°C (cryostate 2800E; Leica, Hamburg, Germany). It is also important to cut at a low speed.

9.4 *IN SITU* HYBRIDIZATION

9.4.1 Serial dilutions and application of probe

After the sections have been cut and equilibrated to hybridization solution in the glass well plates, they are carefully flattened out to remove folds, wrinkles and trapped air bubbles. Care should be taken to immerse sections completely during all steps of the procedure. Partial drying dramatically increases the background. The amount of hybridization solution necessary for covering a free-floating section depends on its size. For coronal adult rat brain sections, about 80 μl is required. For a section through one hemisphere of an adult cat, 120–150 μl may be needed. The plate is covered with the lid and prehybridization performed for 3–4 h at 42–45°C in an oven.

Hybridization times should be determined empirically. We usually prepare the sections on day 1, apply the probes in the evening, and hybridize for 12–16 h, i.e. basically overnight. Washing is carried out on day 2.

Longer times may be necessary when low-level mRNAs must be detected. A convenient time-table is to cut the sections on day 1, and store them overnight in prehybridization solution at −20°C, preferably already sorted into the well plates. Early morning on day 2 the plates should be placed at 42–45°C for 4 h and the probe should be applied by noon. Washing is carried out around noon on day 3.

Sections or cultures stored in prehybridization

Protocol 9.6

1. Thaw out the cRNA probes in ice or by brief incubation at 37°C.
2. Vortex probe and spin down.
3. Prepare serial dilutions in hybridization solution.
4. Vortex vigorously, incubate at 65°C for 5 min (optional), vortex again and spin down.

The optimal dilution depends primarily on the titre of the probe. A transcription of 1 µg of template DNA may yield about 10 µg of riboprobe dissolved in 100 µl of TER. When a stock concentration of 100 ng µl^{-1} is assumed, a dilution of 1:2000 means 5 ng of probe per 80 µl incubation. One transcription would then be sufficient for hybridization of 2000 tissue sections. If, on Northern-blot analysis of the cRNA probe, a clear band is seen, start with a dilution of 1:300 (Figure 9.1, lanes 1,2,4). If a stronger band develops, start with 1:500 (Figure 9.1, lane 3). In the case of very intense bands, such as in lane 5 of Figure 9.1, probes can be diluted up to 1:2000. This probe yields good signals when diluted 1:5000. We have recently carried out a serial dilution (1:300–1:2000) with a riboprobe specific for neuropeptide Y (NPY) mRNA, expressed in a subset of interneurons, in whole-mount organotypic cultures of rat cerebral cortex. We found virtually no difference in specific labelling. The overall background, however, became lower in sections incubated with increasing probe dilution. The optimal dilution has to be determined empirically. It also depends on probe size, how many cells express the target mRNA, how many copies are contained in each cell body, the quality of the tissue, and how stringent the hybridization and the washes can be performed. Probes that are too concentrated will yield a poor background (hybridization to every cell).

Under routine conditions, we therefore use the optimal dilution, if a large series of sections have to be analysed. When subsequent double-labelling experiments are to be carried out, however, we incubate alternate sections in three different dilutions (e.g. 1:500, 1:1000 and 1:1500). The lowest dilution is expected to reveal all mRNA-expressing neurons. However, the staining intensity may be too high in a number of neurons to perform an immunofluorescence, as too much accumulated reaction product may hinder antibody penetration or may quench the fluorescence. The colour development in the sections incubated with the higher probe dilution is carefully monitored. It may result in a lower amount of reaction product (to develop in a given time), and could be stopped when a clear signal is obtained in the neuronal population of interest.

5. For the hybridization, remove glass well plates from the oven, remove the lid.
6. With pipette tips, remove the prehybridization solution, and apply the hybridization solution (the diluted probes).
7. Take care to cover the sections completely from above and below. The sections must be freely floating in the solution.
8. Trapped air bubbles and wrinkles have to be carefully removed. Use yellow pipette tips for this purpose. Do not be afraid of manipulating sections this way. Well-fixed and well-cut sections are quite stable (try to disrupt one), but nevertheless you should avoid poking holes in the structures of interest.
9. Cover plate with lid and place at 42–45°C in an oven.
10. When hybridization is performed in glass vials, pipette off the prehybridization solution and apply the probe.
11. 'Mix' probe solution and sections by swirling; check that sections are floating.
12. Seal vials with parafilm, then cover with a piece of aluminium foil in case parafilm cracks during hybridization.

Protocol 9.7

1. Prepare the washing solutions and equilibrate at hybridization temperature or slightly higher (up to 55°C).
2. Remove plates from the oven.
3. With a brush, fish the sections out of the wells and place into insets/trays (see equipment) in 2 × SSC at room temperature.
4. Rinse briefly.
5. Transfer to prewarmed 2 × SSC and wash for 15 min at 42–55°C.
6. Continue washing in prewarmed 2 × SSC/50% formamide, 0.1 × SSC/50% formamide, and 0.1 × SSC (15 min each wash). This means that sections have to remain for 15 min at the chosen temperature! Wash temperature and duration can be varied. Try higher temperatures (50–55°C) or prolonged washes if the background is too high even though the probe is sufficiently diluted.
7. After the last wash, transfer to 1 × TBS or buffer DIG-I at room temperature and equilibrate in three changes for about 15 min.

solution can be started at any time. Tubes are warmed to room temperature, the desired amount of section is removed with a sterile glass hook into the glass wall plates; prehybridization is carried out for another 1 or 2 h. The probes are then applied.

9.4.2. Washing the sections

After the hybridization, sterility is no longer necessary. From now on sections can be handled with histology equipment, i.e. artist's brushes, normal laboratory dishes simply cleaned in a dish washer and without gloves.

9.4.3 Immunodetection of hybrid molecules

The procedure requires blocking, antibody incubation, washes and colour detection. Sections must be prevented from drying throughout the procedure. The blocking reagent comes from Boehringer, but could be replaced by a 1–5% BSA solution.

Note, that the AP reaction products are formazan salts, which are not particularly stable in ethanol and xylene-based media. So do not try long-term storage of sections. The reaction product may degrade. As an alternative to xylene, use water-soluble mounting media (e.g. Aquatex, Merck) or a home-made medium

(10 mM Tris/HCl, pH 7.5, 10% glycerol and 0.5% gelatine, which buffers, and clears the sections, and binds coverslips to the slides respectively). However, the quality of the sections tends to decline. We therefore recommend analysis of the sections as soon as possible.

9.4.3.1 Results

Results of the ISH procedure are shown in Figure 9.2. The mRNA-expressing neurons can be clearly identified at low power (Figure 9.2a) and higher magnification (Figure 9.2b,c). Neurons of different sizes were labelled. Figure 9.2(c) was taken from a developing rat cortex. Whereas some neurons are well differentiated and express glumatic acid decarboxylase (GAD) mRNA abundantly, others still display immature features and express less GAD mRNA.

Entire sections may be directly printed with a photographic enlarger to chart mRNA-expressing neurons. Figure 9.3(a,b) shows hemispheres of rat cortex at two anterior–posterior levels. GAD mRNA-expressing neurons appear as white dots. In Figure 9.3(a), intensely labelled neurons are present in the septal and basal forebrain area, while the striatum expresses a lower intensity. The cortex expresses mRNA at a moderate intensity. In Figure 9.3(b), the reticular formation of the thalamus is intensely labelled, as is the amydala complex and dorsal hypothalamus. Also the hippocampus contains many intensely

Protocol 9.8

1. While sections are in the hot washes, thaw out an aliquot of 5× blocking solution.
2. Dilute to 1× with DIG-I. Place at 65°C. Vortex to make sure it is completely dissolved. The solution remains turbid, but there should be no visible particles.
3. Carefully clean the glass well plate (dish-washing reagent, long rinse with distilled water, allow to dry).
4. With brushes, transfer sections from DIG-I into blocking solution in the glass well plate. Use about 150 µl per well.
5. Block for 1 h at room temperature.
6. Dilute antibody (AP-labelled sheep-anti-DIG, F(ab)$_2$ fragments) 1:1500 or 1:2000 in DIG-I.
7. Pipette off blocking solution, and rinse sections in the glass wells briefly in DIG-I.
8. Remove DIG-I and apply the antibody to the sections.
9. Cover plate with the lid and incubate for 2 h at room temperature.
10. Transfer sections to DIG-I and rinse 3 × 15 min at room temperature.
11. Clean the glass well plate carefully (the substrate solution may precipitate, if in contact with dirty glassware).
12. Equilibrate sections to pH 9.5 in two changes of TBS/Mg^{2+} buffer, pH 9.5, for 5 min.
13. In a 15 ml polypropylene tube (or clean glass vial) make up substrate solution (always fresh) in TBS/Mg^{2+} buffer. The AP substrates are NBT salt and BCIP. Per 10 ml of TBS/Mg^{2+}, pH 9.5, use 45 µl of NBT stock and 35 µl of BCIP stock (section 2, Table 1). Vortex to mix.
14. Transfer sections to the glass well plate and incubate in about 120 µl of substrate solution. Take care to immerse the sections completely. Incubate in the dark, because the substrate solution is light sensitive. Sections will turn slightly blue/purple after some hours. The colour reaction should then be monitored once in a while by simply placing the glass plate on the stage of a microscope. With low magnification, specifically labelled cells (blue reaction product) should be visible. A good quality probe should give labelled cells within 4–5 h.
15. If it is late in the day, the sections can be stored in substrate solution overnight at +4°C. The reaction will proceed more slowly. Alternatively dilute the substrate solution (try 1:1 dilution with TBS/Mg^{2+} buffer). Check the sections next morning, and continue colour development at room temperature. Mount a section in Tris/Mg^{2+} buffer, monitor with microscope when still wet, transfer back to substrate solution if staining is too weak.
16. Continue the colour reaction until sufficient reaction product has developed in the neurons of interest (check with microscope).
17. Stop the reaction by transferring the sections to Tris/HCl buffer, pH 7.5. Lowering the pH and removal of Mg^{2+} as cofactor inhibits the AP.
18. Rinse 3 × 15 min in Tris/HCl buffer at room temperature.
19. Mount sections on gelatinized slides and air-dry.
20. Store dry in dark slide box.
21. Before analysis, clear by brief dips in ethanol, xylene and coverslip with Eukitt or other mounting medium. Analyze immediately.

Figure 9.2 Results of ISH on brain tissue. (a) GAD mRNA-expressing neurons in cat visual cortex occur in layers I–VI including the white matter below layer VI. (b) Intensely labelled cells at higher magnification. The cytoplasm contains the reaction product, the nucleus is free. (c) Besides a large intensely mRNA-expressing cell resides a small differentiating neuron which starts NPY mRNA expression in cat visual cortex. This finding corresponds well to immunohistochemical data (Wahle & Meyer, 1987). (d,e,f) Cat visual cortex supragranular layers. GAD mRNA-expressing neurons (d) co-express parvalbumin-immunoreactive material (e). The large soma (arrow), which intensely expresses GAD mRNA and also paralbumin, is labelled by fluorescein isothiocyanate (FITC)-conjugated *Vicia villosa* lectin (f). These markers characterize the neurons of a large basket cell.

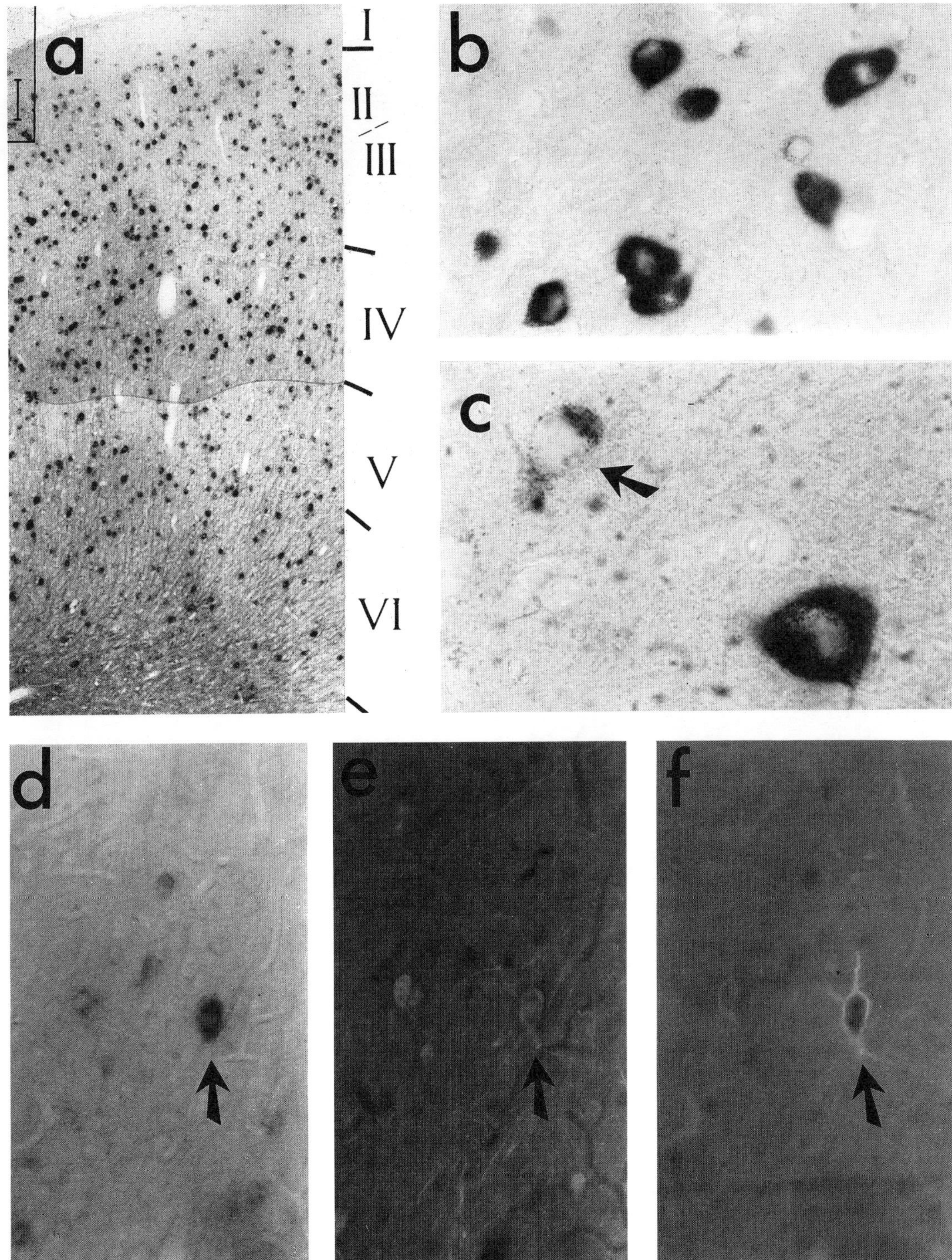

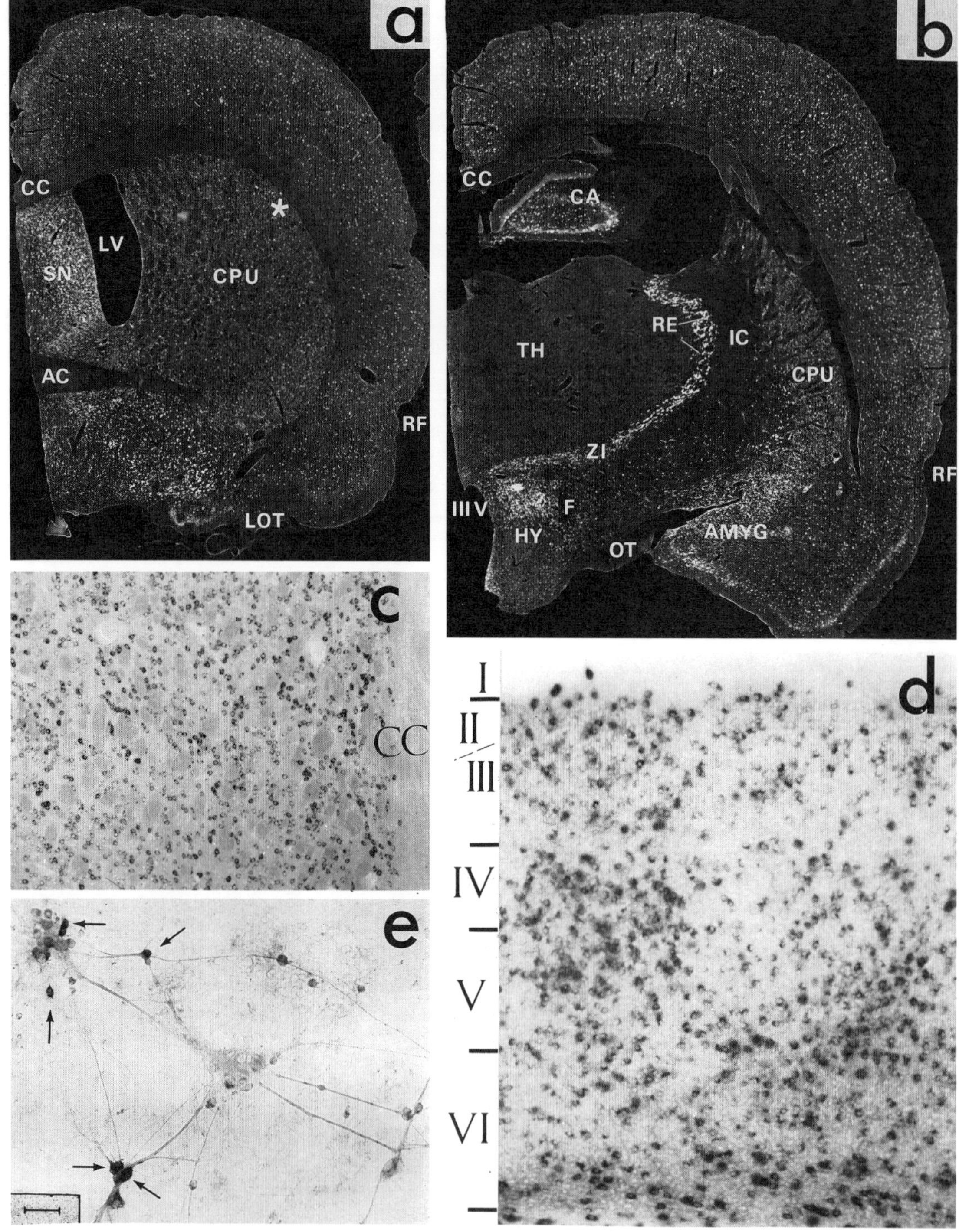
a
CC
LV
SN
CPU
*
AC
RF
LOT
b
CC
CA
TH
RE
IC
CPU
ZI
IIIV
RE
F
HY
OT
AMYG
RF
c
CC
d
I
II
III
IV
V
VI
e

labelled cells intermingled in pyramidal and granule cell layers. Note that this section has handling artefacts. Hippocampus and striatum were disrupted from the corpus callosum. Such artefacts can be avoided by more careful handling of the sections. Arranging the pieces properly during mounting might also have salvaged some damage.

A closer view of striatal tissue is presented in Figure 9.3(c). Intensely and moderately β-preprotachykinin mRNA-expressing spiny stellate cells are shown.

The hypothalamus contained intensely GAD mRNA-expressing cells *in vivo* (Figure 9.3b) and also *in vitro* (Figure 9.3e; from Wahle *et al.*, 1993). Dissociated embryonic day-13 rat hypothalamus cells had been cultured for 4 weeks. GAD mRNA-expressing neurons (arrows) can be clearly delineated from unstained cells in this phase-contrast photomicrograph (unstained cells appear grey).

An organotypic culture of rat visual cortex, hybridized *in toto*, is shown in Figure 9.3(d). As *in vivo* (Figure 9.3a,b), many GAD mRNA-expressing neurons can be identified, and different labelling intensities are present. GAD neurons occur in all layers, typically layer I. Clusters of GAD neurons may appear in tissue areas not optimally flattened to a monolayer. ISH for NPY mRNA in these cultures results in a much smaller subset of labelled neurons (see Colour Plate 3).

9.4.4. Counterstaining the sections

As formazan reaction products are not very stable in ethanol and xylene, the normal histological procedure of counterstaining, for instance with thionin (which stains the 'Nissl substance' in endoplasmic reticulum) cannot be performed, because it requires prolonged exposure to differentiating ethanols. Also, the Nissl substance is where the AP reaction product has developed. Several histological techniques are incompatible with immediate counterstaining, for instance some fluorescent tracers, some benzidine reaction products, and also radioactive hybridizations. Here, prolonged exposure to ethanol bleaches the reduced silver grains in dipped sections resulting in a loss of signal. Therefore one would usually evaluate the ISH reaction first, and then counterstain selected sections, to obtain information about area boundaries and cortical layers.

Another method is counterstaining with fluorescent dyes. The sections should be immersed in diamidinophenylindole (DAPI) 0.002% (Sigma) in phosphate buffer for several minutes followed by three washes in phosphate buffer. DAPI binds to nuclear chromatin and gives an intense blue fluorescence under UV excitation. It allows one to distinguish neuronal from glial cells by nuclear morphology (see below), and also gives a fair picture of cortical layers and CNS areas. It is stable even when coverslipped with xylene-based media.

9.4.5 Troubleshooting the staining procedure

Besides probe and tissue quality, we had little problem obtaining good ISH signals. Optimal dilution is critical for a good signal-to-noise ratio, and has to be determined empirically. As Wisden and Morris pointed out (Chapter 1), most of the pretreatments are unnecessary for brain tissue. Only PK, by digesting proteins, enhances signal intensity due to exposure of target mRNA. All

Figure 9.3 ISH stained sections printed with a photographic enlarger. (a) Frontal section through rat telencephalic centres. (b) Section through the diencephalon. The mRNA-expressing cells appear as white dots. Cell density and intensity of mRNA expression can be compared between the structures. (c): Higher magnification of rat striatum (corresponds to the area marked with an asterisk in (a)) in an alternating section revealing β-preprotachykinin mRNA-expressing neurons. (d) GAD mRNA expression in neurons in organotypic cultures of rat visual cortex. Cells occur in all layers (indicated). (e) GAD mRNA expression in dissociated cultures (phase contrast). Arrows indicate GAD neurons. Other cell somata do not contain the dark-blue reaction product. **Abbreviations**: AC, anterior commissure; AMYG, amygdala; CA, cornu ammonis of hippocampus; CC, corpus callosum; CPU, caudate putamen; IC, internal capsule; F, fornix; HY, hypothalamus; LOT, lateral olfactory tract; LV, lateral ventrical; OT, optic tract; RE, thalamic reticular formation; RF, rhinal fissure; TH, thalamus; ZI, zona incerta; III V, third ventricle.

Protocol 9.9

Equipment: To rinse sections we use plastic staining trays with fitted Plexiglass plate insets which have regularly spaced holes (can be made by most machine shops). One side of the plate is covered with a nylon mesh (can be glued to the Plexiglass). These plates are used for washing sections. Preferably, the matrix of holes in the Plexiglass plates is arranged such that it corresponds to the matrix of wells in the glass well plates of tissue culture plates used for hybridization. Our glass well plates have 30 wells (6 by 5). The Plexiglass plates have 72 wells (6 by 12), so the sections of two glass well plates can be rinsed in one Plexiglass plate. Further requirements are fine artist's brushes and gelatinized slides.
Reagents: as in Sections 9.2 and 9.3.
Solutions:
20×SSC (Section 9.3) is diluted to 2× and 0.1× with double-distilled water. Do not autoclave.
2×SSC/50% formamide: Mix 2 × SSC 1:1 with formamide (straight from the bottle).
0.1×SSC/50% formamide: Mix 0.1 × SSC 1:1 with formamide.
10×Tris/HCl (0.5 M): 121 g of Tris dissolved in 300 ml of distilled water, brought to pH 7.5 with 740 ml 1 M HCl. Fill up to 2 litres with distilled water.

pretreatments, however, reduce tissue quality, and, in particular, free-floating sections tend to stick to brushes and equipment. Pretreatments may also destroy cell marker molecules or expose unwanted epitopes, which was our main reason for omitting these steps. RNAases have so far not been a problem in ISH. After the perfusion, the tissue is soaked with formaldehyde, which effectively denatures protein. The cryoprotection solution is made with DEPC-treated buffer and RNAase-free sucrose, and sterile tools are used for handling. We use OTC compound (TissueTek, Miles) for embedding. Equipment (cryostate, Plexiglass blade, knife) is cleaned with SDS and ethanol, sterile tools are used for cutting, and, soon after cutting, the sections are in a formamide-containing solution, which again inhibits RNAases. Post-hybridization washes and detection are carried out in non-sterile laboratory dishes. We have seen no necessity for RNAase A post-treatment, as the reactions have yielded a high specificity. The anti-DIG antibody in a concentrated form is stable; so far, we have never had reason to believe that failure of an ISH was due to failure of the antibody/enzyme. The enzyme can be checked by running the labelled control cRNA on a gel and detecting the band by Northern blotting. To check the enzyme, 0.5 µl of antibody is spotted on to nitrocellulose and run in an AP reaction. The blue spot indicates that the enzyme is working. It is important to ensure that the pH of the AP reaction is optimal, and the substrates are mixed in the right concentrations.

9.5 IMMUNOHISTOCHEMISTRY

9.5.1 Antibodies compatible with the protocol

Protocol 9.10 is a short version of our routine immunohistochemistry protocol.

We have successfully tested a variety of combinations: NPY mRNA and NPY immunofluorescence, GAD mRNA and neuropeptide (NPY or somatostatin) immunofluorescence, substance P mRNA and somatostatin immunofluorescence, neuropeptide or GAD mRNA and antibodies against structural proteins (microtubule-associated protein MAP2, or neurofilaments or Alzheimer precursor protein; Boehringer), calcium-binding protein (parvalbumin) and others. Examples for double-labelled cells are shown in Colour Plate 3(f,g). Here,

Protocol 9.10

1. Stop the colour development in 1×Tris/HCl buffer, pH 7.5. Do not allow sections to dry; it is best to proceed directly to the immunohistochemistry.
2. Rinse 3×15 min in 1×TBS at room temperature.
3. Block sections in 1–5% BSA in TBS for 30 min at room temperature. Alternatively, use normal animal serum for blocking (e.g. normal goat serum 3% in TBS). Make sure that further antibodies of the immune cascade do not cross-react with the blocking serum, or with the sheep anti-DIG antibody.
4. Transfer sections to the primary antibody at working dilution (depends on antibody titre and antigen to be detected and has to be determined on control sections made from the same tissue block).
5. Incubate for 12–16 h or longer at +4°C (depends on the antigen, and has to be determined on control sections).
6. Rinse sections 3 × 15 min in TBS.
7. Transfer to secondary antibody usually diluted according to the manufacturer's recommendation.
8. Incubate for 2–4 h at room temperature (or longer at +4°C).
9. Rinse sections 3 × 15 min in TBS.
10. If the secondary antibody is conjugated to fluorochrome, mount sections and coverslip, when still moist, with TBS-buffered glycerol (mixed 1:1). Seal coverslip to the slide with nail polish; this prevents evaporation of mounting medium (make sure that nail polish has no autofluorescence). Analyse immediately.
11. If an immunoperoxidase reaction is carried out, incubate in tertiary antibody (enzyme-tagged complex, horseradish peroxidase (HRP) at working dilution for 2–4 h at room temperature.
12. Rinse sections 3 × 15 min in TBS.
13. Develop the HRP reaction product with diaminobenzidine (DAB) as chromogen. Make up 0.02–0.03% DAB in Tris/HCl, pH 7.5. Dissolve completely. Note that benzidines are suspected carcinogens.
14. Preincubate sections in DAB solution for 5–10 min at room temperature (in the dark).
15. Add H_2O_2 as substrate for the peroxidase to a final concentration of 0.003%. Incubate for 5 min at room temperature. Sections turn light brown.
16. Stop the reaction by transferring sections to rinse buffer (Tris/HCl, pH 7.5), rinse several times and mount on gelatinized slides. Air-dry sections. Coverslip with xylene-based or watery mounting medium and analyse.

NPY mRNA-expressing neurons in an organotypic culture of rat visual cortex co-express NPY-immunoreactive material. In Figure 9.2(d,e,f), triple-labelling is shown. A large basket neuron in the adult cat visual cortex was identified by expressing GAD mRNA (Figure 9.2d), parvalbumin-immunoreactive material (Figure 9.2e) and a lectin-binding site (Figure 9.2f) on the cell's outer membrane (see Section 9.5.3).

So far, all antibodies that exhibited staining on control sections of a tissue block also exhibited staining of virtually equal intensity on alternate sections processed for ISH. The initial perfusion fixation is the most important factor for antigen preservation in brain tissue. Most antigens currently under investigation are intracellular antigens which could be well fixed with a paraformaldehyde perfusion. We have not tested antibodies to fragile extracellular membrane-bound epitopes (e.g. gangliosides). We do not know if such epitopes survive ISH, but we know that lectin-binding sites, for instance, do (Section 9.5.3).

Detection of antigens requiring a high percentage of glutardialdehyde in the fixative (e.g. amino acid transmitters γ-aminobutyrate (GABA) or glutamate) is less compatible with the above ISH protocol, because the procedure tolerates only small amounts of glutardialdehyde. A higher percentage of this fixative strongly cross-links the tissue such that probe penetration becomes less effective. Borohydrate or proteinase K pretreatment may be used to overcome this effect, but the small amino acid transmitter molecules may be lost during these steps. Effects on mRNA retention have to be evaluated.

9.5.2 Secondaries and labelling reaction

Secondary and tertiary antibodies depend on the type of labelling reaction to be carried out. Fluorescence-tagged secondaries are usually obtained from Dakopatts, Hamburg, Germany or Molecular Probes, USA, and are diluted according to the manufacturer's recommendation. The optimal dilution (signal versus background) must be determined on the tissue of interest.

Indirect immunofluorescence is performed quickly and can be analysed immediately. An immunoperoxidase reaction requires more time. Both peroxidase–anti-peroxidase (PAP, from Dakopatts) reaction and avidin–biotin–HRP (ABC reagent from Dakopatts or Vector Labs) reaction can be carried out. For the PAP reaction, an affinity-purified secondary antibody against the primary antibody is applied. PAP complex is composed of antibodies from the species delivering the primary antibody (for example, primary is a polyclonal serum raised in rabbit, secondary is a goat anti-rabbit serum, tertiary is rabbit PAP).

The ABC reaction is another three-step procedure. The secondary is an affinity-purified antibody against the primary and is tagged with biotin. The ABC reagent has two components, avidin or streptavidin and biotin tagged with an enzyme, usually HRP. The two components are titred together such that the resulting complex has free binding sites for the biotin tagged to the secondary (the manufacturer's recommendation should be followed).

The enzyme for the colorimetric detection is usually HRP, and the chromogen is DAB. HRP destroys peroxides such as H_2O_2 to H_2O and O_2. Emitted electrons cause polymerization of the DAB to a brown product. The critical parameter is the concentration of H_2O_2. It should be kept low (max. 0.005% final concentration); 150 µl per 200 ml of DAB reaction volume should be added from a prediluted (1% in H_2O, always prepared fresh) stock slowly into the solution. Stir to mix. Too much H_2O_2 causes a high background. As with different substrates for the AP, other chromogens in an HRP reaction give differently coloured reaction products. The DAB reaction product is brown and stable. Sections can be viewed with a light microscope, and structural details can be much more easily analysed than with fluorescence. If the reaction product is light brown, the darker blue of the AP reaction product is easily detectable. However, depending on the amount of antigen in the target cell, the somata may be dark brown. Then, it becomes hard to detect a smaller amount of AP reaction product. Also, expensive colour pictures are needed for documentation, whereas fluorescence can be photographed on black and white film.

9.5.3 Histochemistry: lectin probes

Plant lectins have been recently introduced into neurobiology. Membrane proteins bind lectins via carbohydrate domains. The expression of membrane proteins and their post-translational modifications are often cell-type specific, and therefore certain lectins stain certain neurons exclusively, often with the selectivity of a monoclonal antibody. In the CNS and the cerebral cortex, lectins label distinct cell types, but not neighbouring cells of other types. They can therefore be used as selective markers of cell types. Lectins are obtained conjugated to enzymes or fluorochromes. We have tried the lectin *Vicia villosa agglutinin* (VVA) conjugated to HRP and to the fluorescent marker FITC (purchased from Medac, Hamburg, Germany; this supplier offers many different lectins conjugated to different markers) in combination with ISH. VVA delineates basically two interneuronal

Protocol 9.11

1. Stop the colour development of the ISH in Tris/HCl buffer, pH 7.5.
2. Rinse sections 3 × 15 min in Tris/HCl.
3. Dilute VVA conjugated to HRP in Tris/HCl to 5 µg ml^{-1} and incubate the sections for 12 h at +4°C.
4. Rinse sections in Tris/HCl.
5. Develop HRP activity with DAB and H_2O_2 (see above). Sections turn light brown.

Protocol 9.12

Equipment: same as in previous sections.
Reagents: H_2O_2 (approx. 30% stock Perhydrol, Merck), DAB (Sigma).
Solutions:
DAB stock: In order to reduce exposure to powdered DAB, make up a 100 × stock solution. Dissolve 2 g of DAB in 100 ml of distilled water (fume hood, gloves). Store 1 ml portions at − 20°C. It is stable for a year. Use 1 aliquot per 100 ml 1× Tris/HCl reaction volume. Laboratory dishes in contact with benzidines are immersed in hypochloride solution to bleach the DAB.

cell types in the cat neocortex, the large basket neurons and neurogliform neurons and stains larger interneurons in the hippocampus. The lectin thus allows identification of these types in the population of GAD mRNA-expressing neurons.

Double-labelled neurons are shown in Colour Plate 3(d,e). They can be identified by a brown reaction product distributed along the cell's outer membrane, often extending far into the dendritic compartment. In the VVA/FITC-labelled material, the cell membrane is fluorescent. In Figure 9.2(d–f) triple labelling is shown. The GAD mRNA was detected in the cytoplasm of a large basket neuron, which was identified by the lectin-binding site (green FITC fluorescence on the membrane) and a calcium-binding protein, parvalbumin (detected in the cytoplasm and dendrites by Texas Red fluorescence). Besides information about a biochemical feature of the neurons (expression of a particular carbohydrate), one also obtains information on the geometry of the dendritic tree, which helps compare the mRNA-expressing neurons with cell types initially described by classical morphological techniques (Golgi impregnation). The presence of parvalbumin is related to a physio-logical feature; these neurons are fast-spiking cells and fire bursts of action potentials (Naegele & Katz, 1990). We assume that other extracellular epitopes are equally stable throughout the ISH, and could be subsequently detected with lectin probes or with monoclonal antibodies.

AP can also be developed with substrates giving a red reaction product (Fast Violet B/Naphthol-AS-E-phosphate, Section 9.2). This results in a red cytoplasmic stain and a brown membrane lining. Results are shown in Colour Plate 3(d) compared with the blue reaction product in Colour Plate 3(e).

9.6 TRACT TRACING

9.6.1 Injection of marker substances

The example presented here is taken from a recent study (Wahle *et al.*, 1993). We attempted to demonstrate whether neurons in the nucleus of the optic tract (NOT) projecting to the lateral geniculate nucleus (LGN) express GAD mRNA. Previous attempts to identify GAD or GABA

immunohistochemically had failed (Nabors &
Mize, 1991).

Adult cats were anaesthetized with ketamine/
Rompun. Body temperature and heart rate were
monitored. A craniotomy was performed to
expose the target area, the LGN. To identify the
LGN, visually evoked activity was recorded with
microelectrodes. After confirming the position,
a Hamilton syringe was lowered through the
electrode tract into the LGN, and rhodamine-
conjugated latex microspheres (beads; Luma
Fluor New City, NY, USA) were injected as a
concentrated solution. The craniotomy was
closed with the bone plate, secured with dental
cement, and the wound was sutured. Antibiotics
and analgesics were administered postoperatively.
Animals survived for 3 days, during which the
axon terminals of NOT neurons in the LGN took
up the beads and transported them back
(retrogradely) towards the somata.

9.6.2 Processing the tissue

Perfusion and tissue processing followed the
protocols given in Sections 9.2 and 9.3. The
midbrain containing the NOT was dissected and
sectioned at 20 μm thickness from the posterior
aspect of the LGN to mid-level superior
colliculus. From each experiment, about 180
cryostat sections were processed serially in well
plates, hybridized to antisense GAD cRNA
probe.

We identified two populations of GAD
mRNA-expressing neurons. The small ones
correspond well to interneurons of the NOT
identified reproducibly by GABA immunohistochemistry. In addition, however, a population of
large neurons was detected, expressing high
amounts of GAD mRNA. These neurons had
not been observed by GABA immunohistochemistry. Quite a number of these neurons
contained the fluorescent beads. An example
is shown in Colour Plate 3(a–c). Thus large
pretecto-geniculate neurons express GAD mRNA
and are thus GABAergic. The result unequivocally
confirms their functional role as inhibitory
neurons, which has been suggested on the basis
of electrophysiology and morphology, but was
under dispute, because attempts to localize the

inhibitory transmitter GABA in the large
neurons had failed in most cases (Nabors and
Mize, 1991). ISH in this particular case has not
simply just revealed a neuronal mRNA. Rather
it has helped to define the role of a particular
CNS cell type functionally modulating (via a
disinhibition) the LGN relay neurons during
saccadic eye movements (M. Schmidt and K.-P.
Hoffmann, unpublished work).

Fluorescent tracers are advantageous, as they
are simply viewed under the microscope. Beads
emit a strong fluorescence. Nevertheless it is
recommended to monitor the colour development of the ISH because, if too much reaction
product accumulates in the neurons, it may
quench the fluorescence. Besides the beads,
fluorogold has been used in combination with
radioactive ISH (Burgunder & Young, 1988).

When enzyme tracers (e.g. HRP) are used,
one must determine whether the activity survives
the hybridization, because tracer detection
should be carried out after the hybridization,
otherwise sections (with mRNA exposed) would
be in a number of different (and hard to sterilize)
substrate solutions and washes for quite some
time. Lectin tracers could probably be used, as
they can be detected with antibodies. Although
we have not tried it, we assume that they behave
like other tissue antigens, which survive the
hybridization.

9.7 ANALYSIS AND PRESENTATION

The AP reaction product, developed with NBT
and BCIP, is amorphous and blue, or black in
heavily mRNA-expressing cells. The reaction
product develops initially around the nucleus,
where the concentration of cellular mRNA
bound to ribosomes and endoplasmic reticulum
is highest. Later, more peripheral parts of the
soma light up, and in several instances, e.g. with
mRNA encoding the substance P receptor and
also with neuropeptide mRNAs, the staining
extends for a considerable distance into the
primary dendrites. If sections have to be analysed
with high magnification, they must be coverslipped with xylene-based media, and will soon
decay. Water-based media allow observation up

to 40× magnification, which is good for most purposes (e.g. analysis of double-labelling). Under higher magnification the view is blurred.

Sections can be analysed with any normal light microscope. Nomarski optics (phase-contrast interference) can be applied. It visualizes for instance the nuclei of the labelled cells, and by nuclear morphology, neurons can be distinguished from glia. Neuronal nuclei are larger, round, or slightly ovally elongated, and display one round nucleolus. Glia nuclei are smaller, sometimes multiform and have one or more quite small nucleoli. When sections are counterstained with DNA-binding dyes (e.g. DAPI), the neuronal nuclei are faintly stained and glial nuclei are more intensely stained as a result of more condensed chromatin, and nucleoli appear as tiny blue dots (this difference helped in the identification of neurons for intracellular injection with Lucifer Yellow) under UV excitation. As the nuclei are void of staining, no reaction product quenches the fluorescence.

Fluorescein, rhodamin and Texas Red, fluorochromes tagged to secondary antibodies or latex beads, are equally well detected in the somata and neurites (Colour Plate 3). In heavily labelled cells, somatic immunofluorescence may be partly quenched by the reaction product, partly because we have frequently observed an inhomogeneous distribution of AP reaction product in the soma. Often it is more concentrated in one somatic pole. Therefore the colour development must be stopped as soon as sufficient reaction product has developed in the soma. Then peripheral parts of the soma and the dendrites can usually be easily visualized by immunofluorescence, which in some cases is brilliant in the somatic pole opposite to the mRNA-containing pole. It suggests that mRNA and peptide product are concentrated in different parts of the cell, a phenomenon explained by the known intracellular processing (translation, peptide trafficking and storage) pathways. Sometimes the nucleus appears 'labelled' in double-labelled cells, because fluorescence shines through the AP-negative nucleus from behind. Double-labelled neurons may therefore display several patterns: fluorescence and mRNA may either co-extend into the same somatic parts, or may be accumulated in different somatic parts, or fluorescent neurites may

arise from an mRNA-positive but fluorescence-negative soma. This accounts also for retrogradely labelled neurons. The beads and the mRNA may co-extend or may be localized in different compartments of the cell, e.g. beads in the dendrites, mRNA in the soma.

The same is true for the homogeneously brown DAB reaction product in immunoperoxidase reactions (see Section 9.5.2). Ideally, double-labelled neurons contain the blue–black amorphous AP reaction product around the nuclei and the brown DAB product in peripheral somatic parts or dendritic/axonal compartments of the neurons. Immunoperoxidase may be the method of choice when longer-living preparations are preferred or no fluorescence photomicroscope is available. It is also easier to reconstruct, e.g., a peptide innervation pattern in the structure of interest, besides analysis of double-labelled cells. Further, immunoperoxidase reaction products can be visualized at the electron-microscopic level. This would allow analysis of the synaptology of identified mRNA-expressing cells. Disadvantages are that the AP reaction product is hard to detect in cells expressing large amounts of, e.g. a peptide antigen, so that the DAB reaction product becomes too dark.

The mRNA-expressing cells are photographed on colour or black and white film (for example, Ilford PanF) and are presented as black and white prints for publication. The distribution of mRNA-expressing cells can be charted with an X/Y plotter attached to the stage of the microscope or any computer-based reconstruction program. Alternatively, the sections (mounted on glass slides and coverslipped) may be placed in a photographic enlarger and printed directly on black and white film (shown in Figure 9.3a,b). This is a fast convenient way to chart mRNA-expressing neurons. For double-labelled cells, it is recommended to photograph any fluorescence first, followed by a mixed exposure (fluorescence excitation wavelength plus brightfield at very low intensity) and then brightfield exposure.

ACKNOWLEDGEMENTS

I wish to thank Drs A. Tobin and D. Kaufman for the GAD cDNA, Dr. D. Larhammar for the rat genomic NPY DNA, and Dr. J. Krause for the β-preprotachykinin cDNA. Kirstin Obst and Kike Gutierrez, students in my laboratory produced some of the results. This work was supported by DFG 'Neurovision' and Boehringer Mannheim.

REFERENCES

Ausubel, F.M., Brent, R., Kingston, R.E., Moore, D.D., Seidman, J.G., Smith, J.A. & Struhl, K. (eds.) (1987) *Current protocols in molecular biology*. Greene Publishing Associates and Wiley-Interscience.

Burgunder J.-M. & Young III, W.S. (1988) *Mol. Brain Res.* **4**, 179–189.

Emson, P.C. (1993) *Trends Neurosci.* **16**, 9–16.

Gähwiler, B.H. (1988) *Trends Neurosci.* **11**, 484–489.

Nabors, L.B. and Mize, R.R. (1991) *J. Neurosci.* **11**, 2460–2476.

Naegele & Katz (1990) *J. Neurosci.* **10**, 540–557.

Sambrook, J., Frisch, E.F. and Maniatis, T. (1989) Molecular Cloning: A laboratory manual, 2nd edn, Cold Spring Harbor Laboratory Press, Cold Spring Harbor, NY.

Swandulla, D. & Misgeld, U. (1990) *J. Neurophysiol.* **64**, 715–726.

Wahle, P. & Beckh, S. (1992) *J. Neurosci. Methods* **41**, 153–166.

Wahle, P. & Meyer, G. (1987) *J. Comp. Neurol.* **261**, 165–193.

Wahle, P., Müller, T. & Swandulla, D. (1993) *Brain Res.*, **611**, 37–45.

Wahle, P., Stuphorn, V., Schmidt, M. & Hoffmann, K.-P. (1994) *Europ. J. Neurosci.*, in press.

CHAPTER TEN

Drosophila central nervous system – Non-radioactive *in situ* hybridization using wholemounts

A. ULTSCH

BASF Ltd, Department of Biotechnology, Carl-Bosch-Str. 38, D-67056 Ludwigshafen, Germany

10.1 INTRODUCTION

A wholemount *in situ* hybridization (ISH) technique employing a digoxygenin-labelled nucleic acid probe for the detection and localization of a segmentation gene transcript in morphologically intact *Drosophila* embryos was first reported by Tautz & Pfeifle (1989). The protocol presented in this chapter is based upon the original method.

The non-radioactive wholemount ISH technique provides an elegant experimental tool for studying the three-dimensional accumulation of gene transcripts within developing *Drosophila* embryos. To address the same scientific question using tissue sections one would have to perform time-consuming embedding and serial sectioning of embryos. Moreover, it is cumbersome to reconstruct the three-dimensional localization of a transcript from serial sections. The fact that a typical non-radioactive ISH experiment can be completed within 2 days gives it an additional edge over radioactive techniques. Some researchers seem to prefer antibody staining to nucleic acid hybridization; the production of a good immune serum, however, takes time, whereas digoxygenin-labelled nucleic acid probes can be generated within a day. This considerably faster availability of a non-radioactive probe compared with antibodies may be a significant advantage when a newly discovered gene or gene fragment is to be quickly characterized with respect to its spatial expression pattern during *Drosophila* embryogenesis.

It is generally believed that non-radioactive *in situ* detection methods are significantly less sensitive than radioactive techniques. However, although *Drosophila* wholemount ISH experiments were originally used for the detection of abundant gene transcripts (Tautz & Pfeifle, 1989), this technique has in recent years been considerably refined with respect to its sensitivity and is now used even on vertebrate embryos. For example, non-radioactive *in situ* localization of low-abundance transcripts has recently been

IN SITU HYBRIDIZATION PROTOCOLS FOR THE BRAIN
ISBN 0–12–759919–3

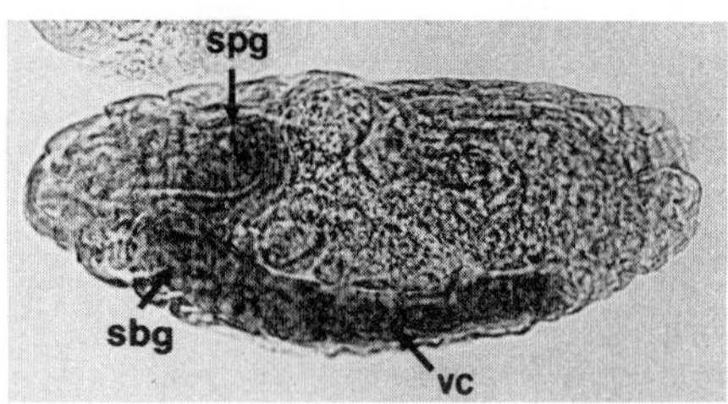

Figure 10.1 Detection by wholemount ISH of mRNA encoding the DGluR-I subunit of glutamate receptors in a late *Drosophila* embryo. ISH was performed on wholemount embryos using a digoxygenin-labelled DGluR-I cDNA fragment (see Ultsch *et al.*, 1992). The lateral view shows specific staining of the developing nervous system; arrows indicate the supra- and sub-oesophageal ganglia (spg and sbg, respectively) and the ventral cord (vc). This figure was taken, with permission, from Ultsch *et al.* (1992).

reported for quail embryos (Coutinho *et al.*, 1992). The sensitivity of this technique has possibly been improved by the use of either *in vitro* transcribed antisense RNA or polymerase chain reaction-generated DNA probes which appear to be characterized by a greater 'specific activity'. In contrast, the original protocol (Tautz & Pfeifle, 1989) employs DNA probes that have been random-primer-labelled with digoxygenin.

An important limitation of the protocol given in this chapter is the fact that its use is restricted to the localization of gene transcripts in *Drosophila* embryos. Wholemount specimens from other developmental stages (e.g. larvae, pupae) are poorly penetrated, if at all, by hybridization probes and require conventional tissue sectioning.

I have used the non-radioactive wholemount hybridization technique to analyse the spatial distribution of *Drosophila* glutamate receptor gene transcripts *in situ* (Ultsch *et al.*, 1992). The result of this analysis is illustrated in Figure 10.1.

10.2 PROTOCOLS

Protocol 10.1 Pretreatment of embryos

1. Collect staged wild-type *Drosophila* embryos from apple juice plates (Ashburner, 1989), rinse briefly with 0.7% NaCl, 0.03% Triton X-100, and dechorionate in 6% sodium hypochlorite for 1–2 min. Rinse as before.
2. Transfer embryos to a 50 ml glass bottle containing 4 ml of the following solution: 100 mM N-(2-hydroxyethyl)piperazine-N'-(2-ethanesulphonic acid (HEPES; pH 6.9 with NaOH), 2 mM $MgSO_4$ and 1 mM ethylene-glycol-bis(2–aminoethyl ether)-N,N,N',N'-tetra-acetic acid (EGTA; pH 8.0).
3. Add 0.5 ml of 37% formaldehyde (Merck, p.a. grade. No pretreatments required; use straight out of the bottle) and 5 ml of heptane.
4. Shake the screw-capped glass bottle vigorously for 15–20 min.
5. Remove and discard lower phase. Add methanol to the upper phase (heptane) in small amounts until embryos sink to the bottom (if embryos are to be stored at this point, replace the methanol with 100% ethanol; embryos may now be stored at −20°C for several weeks).
6. Transfer an aliquot of embryos (300–400 µl) into a 1.5 ml Eppendorf tube. Wash embryos in 1 ml of methanol and then in 1 ml of a solution consisting of methanol, PBT^a, 37% formaldehyde (50:45:5, by vol.).
7. Fix embryos in 1 ml of PBT/37% formaldehyde (95:5, v/v) for 20 min.
8. Wash embryos three times in 1 ml of PBT for 2 min.
9. Split embryos into 50 µl aliquots and transfer these into 650 µl test tubes; siliconize and autoclave test tubes before use.

10. Add 0.5 ml of proteinase K (Merck; 50 mg ml^{-1} of PBS) to each test tube.
11. Incubate three embryo aliquots for 3, 4 and 5 min. Optimal incubation times have to be determined empirically; however, one of the incubation times recommended here should yield satisfactory results. **Note**: overdigestion with proteinase K leads to disintegration of embryos. Therefore, check a few embryos after proteinase K treatment under a low-power light microscope.
12. Inhibit proteinase K by washing the embryos, initially twice in 0.5 ml of a glycine solution (2 mg of glycine/ml of PBT), followed by two washes in 0.5 ml of PBT.
13. Fix embryos as before (step 7).
14. Finally, wash embryos five times in 0.5 ml of PBT for 2 min.

[a] PBT is 1 × PBS + 0.1% Tween 20. 1 × PBS consists of 80 mM Na$_2$HPO$_4$, 20 mM NaH$_2$PO$_4$, 130 mM NaCl, pH 7.2. **Note**: Make up PBS using diethyl pyrocarbonate (DEPC)-treated *aqua dest.* (40 µl of DEPC per 1000 ml of *aqua dest.*) and autoclave. DEPC is supplied by Sigma.

Protocol 10.2 Probe labelling

DNA probes were random hexamer-primer labelled with digoxygenin-11-dUTP using the 'DIG DNA Labeling and Detection Kit' from Boehringer Mannheim.

1. Mix x µl of linearized, freshly denatured[a] DNA (100–2000 ng)
     2 µl of hexanucleotide mixture[b]
     2 µl of dNTP labelling mixture[b]
     y µl of sterile H$_2$O ($y = 19 - x - 4$)
     1 µl of Klenow enzyme (2 units)[b]
2. Incubate for 15–20 h at 37°C.

The probe can now be used for hybridization (see Protocol 10.3) without further purification. To test the labelling efficiency and probe specificity it is recommended that the DIG-labelled DNA be used in a dot-blot hybridization experiment before being used for wholemount ISH. A good DIG-labelled probe should detect 1 pg of homologous DNA in a dot-blot hybridization experiment. Store probe at −20°C.

[a] Denature DNA by heating in a boiling waterbath for 10 min and quickly chilling on a mixture of ice and NaCl.
[b] This component is contained in the 'DIG DNA Labeling and Detection Kit' supplied by Boehringer Mannheim.

Protocol 10.3 Hybridization

1. Make up the hybridization mixture (HM) consisting of 50% deionized formamide (Fluka), 5 × SSC (1 × SSC: 150 mM NaCl, 15 mM sodium citrate, pH 7.0, with HCl), 100 mg ml^{-1} sonicated and heat-denatured salmon sperm DNA, 100 mg ml^{-1} heat-denatured *Escherichia coli* tRNA, 50 mg ml^{-1} heparin, 0.1% Tween 20. Store HM at −20°C.
2. Transfer 50 µl aliquots of pretreated *Drosophila* embryos (Protocol 10.1) into 650 µl of siliconized and autoclaved test tubes.
3. Wash embryos in HM/PBT (1:1, by vol.) for 10 min and then in HM again for 10 min. Use an orbital shaker (horizontal plane) for this.

4. Prehybridize embryos in 500 μl of fresh HM for 120 min at 45°C.
5. Aspirate off the supernatant and bring total volume to 90 μl with HM.
6. Add 10 μl of DIG-labelled (see Protocol 10.2), heat-denatured DNA probe (about 1 mg ml^{-1}); the probe concentration is estimated on the basis of the amount of probe originally subjected to the DIG-labelling reaction.
7. Hybridize overnight at 45°C in a waterbath. Briefly invert the tubes every 30 min during the first 4 h of incubation.

Protocol 10.4 Post-hybridization washing of embryos

All washings are performed at 45°C in 1 ml of the solutions given below. Use an orbital shaker for all washings.

1. Wash embryos in HM/PBT (1:1, by vol.) for 20 min.
2. Wash embryos in PBT for 20 min.
3. Repeat step 2 four times.

Protocol 10.5 Immunodetection of hybridization events

Use an orbital shaker (horizontal platform) for steps 1–4. All incubations are performed at room temperature.

1. Incubate embryos in 500 μl of preadsorbed, phosphatase-conjugated anti-digoxygenin antibody solution (Boehringer Mannheim) for 120 min. The preadsorption procedure is detailed in Protocol 10.6.
2. Wash embryos in PBT for 20 min.
3. Repeat step 2 three times.
4. Incubate embryos twice for 2 min in signal detection buffer (SDB[a]).
5. Aspirate off SDB.
6. Add 500 μl of SDB containing the colour substrates for the alkaline phosphatase reaction[b] and transfer this into a small glass Petri dish.
7. Add 500 μl of SDB containing colour substrates[b].
8. Let colour develop for 10–90 min in the dark. Colour development may be monitored by viewing a few embryos under a binocular microscope every 10 min.
9. Stop colour development by washing the embryos in PBT.
10. Dehydrate embryos in an ascending ethanol series and store embryos in 100% ethanol at 4°C overnight; the latter treatment results in an enhanced bluish–violet colour.
11. Mount embryos using the 'JB-4 Embedding Kit' supplied by Polysciences Inc. (Warrington, PA, USA; Cat. No. 0226. Follow the protocol contained in the kit).

[a] SDB is 100 mM NaCl, 50 mM Tris/HCl, pH 9.5; 0.1% Tween 20, 1 mM levamisole; levamisole was purchased from Sigma (L 9756).
[b] 4.5 μl of 4-nitroblue tetrazolium chloride (NBT) and 3.5 μl of 5-bromo-4-chloro-2-indolyl-phosphate (X-phosphate) per ml of SDB; NBT and X-phosphate can be obtained from Boehringer Mannheim.

Protocol 10.6 Preadsorption of anti-digoxygenin antibodies

Use an orbital shaker for all subsequent steps which are performed at room temperature.

1. Rehydrate 300 μl of pretreated *Drosophila* embryos (Protocol 10.1, steps 1–5) in a descending ethanol series.
2. Fix embryos in PBT/37% formaldehyde (95:5, v/v) for 15 min.
3. Rinse embryos briefly in PBT.
4. Incubate embryos for 60 min in 0.1% bovine serum albumin (BSA)/ 0.2% Tween 20/0.1 × BBS[a].
5. Wash embryos briefly in PBT.
6. Incubate embryos for 120 min with phosphatase-conjugated, anti-digoxygenin antibody (Boehringer-Mannheim) which has been diluted 1:400 with PBT.
7. Transfer preadsorbed antibody to a fresh test tube and dilute 1:5 with PBT. The antibody can now be used for immunodetection of hybridization events (Protocol 10.5).

[a] 1 × BBS is 38 mM NaCl, 53 mM KCl, 12 mM $MgSO_4$, 6 mM $CaCl_2$, 20 mM glucose, 50 mM saccharose, 0.2% bovine serum albumin (BSA), 10 mM *N*-tris(hydroxymethyl)methyl-glycine (TRICINE; Sigma, T 0377); pH 6.95. Sterilize by filtration. BBS can be stored at −20°C.

ACKNOWLEDGEMENTS

The author wishes to express his gratitude to Professor Heinrich Betz for his interest in the work described in this chapter. The author held a predoctoral fellowship from the Boehringer Ingelheim Fonds (Germany).

REFERENCES

Ashburner, M. (1989) *Drosophila – a laboratory manual*. Cold Spring Harbor Laboratory Press, Cold Spring Harbor, NY.

Coutinho, L.L., Morris, J. & Ivarie, R. (1992) *Biotechniques* **13**, 722–724.

Tautz, D. & Pfeifle, C. (1989) *Chromosoma* **98**, 81–85.

Ultsch, A., Schuster, C.-M., Laube, B., Schloss, P., Schmitt, B. & Betz, H. (1992) *Proc. Natl. Acad. Sci. USA* **89**, 10484–10488.

Index